What students are saying:

"I was accepted to 5 out of 6! - F. Edward Herbert School of Medicine - University of Vermont College of Medicine - Cooper Medical School of Rowan University - Oakland University of William Beaumont School of Medicine - Rutgers Robert Wood Johnson Medical School." – Ada

"Their CASPer prep was really good and showed me obvious things I would have never even thought about before speaking with a consultant. Would highly recommend if your top med schools require this test!"– Joe

"I got accepted to UC Davis, Georgetown, UC Riverside (full scholarship - matriculating), Loma Linda, and UCLA. I've thus far recommended your site to anyone I meet." – Marysia

"Just wanted to drop you a line and let you know that I was accepted into all three schools (Queen's, Mac and U of T) but will be accepting U of T. Thanks again for all the help in the process [application review, CASPer prep & interview prep] and I look forward to seeing you around campus / hospitals in the near future. Cheers," – Sameer

"Hello, the interviews went great, thanks again for all the help [with CASPer & interview prep]! I was accepted to McMaster, Queen's, and NOSM [medical schools]. Thanks again," – Jesse

"Thank you for your assistance in preparing me with the CASPer and MMI interviews! I wanted to let you know that I was accepted at Robert

George.Ramos@mgill.ca

Wood Johnson Medical School! Please extend my thanks to the instructors who helped me prepare. Thanks again," – Jason

"I was accepted to the University of Vermont (UVM) and Quinnipiac (Frank H. Netter MD School of Medicine at Quinnipiac University) and will be going to UVM in the fall, which I'm very excited about! I appreciate all the help BeMo provided me in preparing for my interview!!" – Danielle

"Thanks for checking in. Yes, the interviews went really well - I got into all the universities I interviewed at (Toronto, McMaster, and Northern)!" – Megan

"I have heard back from all the schools I applied to. I was accepted at 6 different veterinary schools: Texas A&M, Midwestern, Mississippi State, Oklahoma State, Penn, and Cornell. I was initially waitlisted at Penn and Cornell. Texas A&M conducted an MMI style interview, while Midwestern, Mississippi State, and Penn had traditional interviews. I will be attending my in-state school, Texas A&M, starting in August. Thank you for all your help!" – Callie

"Thanks for the message. The application process went really well, and I am excited to be attending Columbia University College of Physicians and Surgeons in the fall. Thank you for your help," – Andy

"Good News! I was accepted to all three medical schools where I interviewed: University of Toronto, University of Ottawa, and Albert Einstein College of Medicine. I have officially accepted my offer to U of T... Thanks again for all your help! I was very pleased with the service I received." – Joanna

"Hello! My interviews went great actually. I was accepted at NYMC and UMass Medical School, both of which had MMI interview format. I will be attending UMass in the fall. Both my mock interviews gave me really good preparation and the interviewers were wonderful! So I certainly owe a lot of credit to BeMo for helping me reach my goals :) I'd be happy to write a testimonial, etc. Thank you," – Nate

"I hope you are well. I've received acceptances from the University of Toronto, University of Saskatchewan, and University of British Columbia and I'm on the waitlisted at the University of Ottawa. I think BeMo definitely helped prepare me! I'm very grateful for those who helped me improve and prepare." – Saloni

"Thank you for your email. I'll be attending UCSD in the fall. Thank you for the support and resources!" – Jessica

BeMo's Ultimate Guide to CASPer® Test Prep

How to Increase Your CASPer SIM Score by 23%
Using the Proven Strategies They
May Not Want You to Know

BeMo Academic Consulting Inc.

ISBN: 1722496762

ISBN 13: 978-1722496760

LIST OF CONTRIBUTING AUTHORS

Dr. Behrouz Moemeni, Ph.D., founder & CEO at BeMo

Ms. Ronza Nissan, M.A., admissions expert & lead trainer

Dr. Andrej Arsovski, Ph.D., admissions expert & senior scientist

Dr. Lauren Prufer, M.D., admissions expert

Dr. Helena Frishtack, M.D., admissions expert

Dr. Karim Wafa, M.D., admissions expert

Dr. Jenifer Truong, M.D., admissions expert

Dr. Kyle Paradis, Ph.D., admissions expert

Contents

Acknowledgements:

We would like to thank our students and their parents for putting their trust in us and giving us the privilege to be part of their journey. You have inspired us and taught us lessons we would not have learned on our own. Thank you for your continued support and for investing in our mission. You are the reason we get up in the morning.

We would like to thank the countless number of admissions deans, directors, officers, pre-health advisors and school counselors who have "unofficially" supported our mission. Thank you for encouraging us and most importantly thank you for making us think critically. We appreciate what you do, and we understand the impossible task you face each and every single day.

A huge thanks to our team members, both past and present. BeMo wouldn't be what it is today without you.

And of course, a huge thanks to our family and friends who have been supportive unconditionally even when we couldn't spend as much time with them because of our obsession with our mission here at BeMo.

Foreword

First, CONGRATULATIONS for making the commitment to educate yourself to become not only a competitive applicant, but also a better person, and as a result a better future professional. The fact that you have purchased this book tells us that you understand the value of continuous learning and self-improvement. The world rewards individuals who continuously seek to educate themselves because "knowledge is power." Before we get into the details, we need to set the record straight about why you should listen to us, what this book is all about, who this book is for, and who it is NOT for, but first a few words from our founder and CEO.

Why I founded BeMo®: Message from BeMo's founder and CEO, Dr. Behrouz Moemeni

Sometimes you must do what's important even if the chances of success are slim to none.

Often students ask me what motivated me to found BeMo and what gets me up in the morning.

The answer for me is rather simple and has remained the same since day one.

I started BeMo with my cofounder, Dr. Mo Bayegan, in 2013 as a company - see why it's called "BeMo" now? - but the duo that came to be BeMo really started when we first met back in high school in 1996 and then later solidified during our undergraduate and graduate training years.

We both felt every student deserves access to higher education, regardless of his or her social status or cultural background, because education is the best way to introduce positive change in our world.

Sadly, I believe most of the current admissions practices, tools and procedures are not necessarily fair, are mostly outdated, and more importantly, remain scientifically unproven. Therefore, in 2013 as Mo and I were finishing our graduate studies, we decided to create BeMo to make sure no one is treated unfairly because of flawed admission practices.

At the time I was finishing my Ph.D. studies in the field of Immunology at the University of Toronto, which was a transformational educational experience. I had the privilege to work with one of the sharpest minds in the field, Dr. Michael Julius. He taught me many things over the years and two lessons stayed with me: 1) the tremendous value of curiosity in scientific or technological innovation to seek the truth rather than confirming one's own opinions 2) whatever you do has to be the reason that gets you up in the morning. I admit that I wasn't the best student he could have had but I had a relatively successful time as a Ph.D. student. I won 19 awards and I was invited to 7 international conferences. I was even offered an unsolicited job before I had defended my thesis. The job offered a secure source of income and I would have been able to start paying my mounting student loan debt but I decided to abandon a career in academia in favor of starting BeMo. Despite the uncertainty, many well-established competitors, and lack of secure source income of I felt - and I still do - that the mission was well worth the risk even if the probability of success seemed infinitely slim. I truly believe what we do here at BeMo adds more value to each of our students' lives than anything else I could have done, and I would not trade it for the world.

Over the years, we have been fortunate enough to help many students and have an amazing and steadily growing team. We really couldn't have done it without them and it's been a privilege to teach with them and learn from them over the years (thanks for sticking with us!).

We are aware that our methods have been controversial in some circles, innovative ideas often are. However, we are confident in our belief - and the scientific literature supports this - that current admissions practices are rife with bias and must be improved.

In fact, in 2017, I founded another independent company called SortSmart®, which has created what I consider to be the fairest, most scientifically sound and cost-effective admission screening tool out there. I invite you to visit SortSmart.io to learn more and tell your university admissions office to bring SortSmart to your school.

In the meantime, while SortSmart is gathering momentum, at BeMo, we will continue to support students just like you to make sure no groups of students are treated unfairly. You can rest assured that there is no stopping us.

To your success,
Behrouz Moemeni, Ph.D.
CEO @ BeMo

Here's A Bit About Us: BeMo Academic Consulting ("BeMo") BeMoAcademicConsulting.com

We're an energetic academic consulting firm, comprised of a team of researchers and professionals, who use a proven evidence-based and scientific approach to help prospective students with career path development and admissions to undergraduate, graduate, and professional programs such as medicine, law, dentistry, and pharmacy.

We believe your education is one of your most valuable assets and learning how to become a great future professional or scholar doesn't need to be complicated. We also believe that every student deserves access to higher education, regardless of his or her social status or cultural background. However, in our opinion, most of the current admissions practices, tools and procedures are not necessarily fair, are often outdated, and more importantly, remain scientifically unproven.

Our goal is to create truly useful (and scientifically sound) programs and tools that work and provide more than just some trivial information like the other "admissions consulting companies" out there. We want to make sure everyone has a fair chance of admission to highly competitive professional programs despite current biased admissions practices.

We do whatever it takes to come up with creative solutions and then implement like mad scientists. We're passionate about mentoring our students. We're obsessed with delivering useful educational programs and we go where others dare not to explore.

Why should you listen to us?

Our primary area of focus is preparation of applicants for extremely competitive professional schools. Specifically, we are the leaders in CASPer preparation, multiple mini interview (MMI) preparation, traditional interview preparation, video interview preparation and application review. We have an exceptional team of practicing professionals, medical doctors, scholars, and scientists who have served as former CASPer raters and admissions committee members (visit our website, BeMoAcademicConsulting.com to learn more about our admissions experts). To give you an idea, each year we help thousands of students gain admission to top schools around the world. What we are about to share is based on what we have learned in our much sought-after one-on-one coaching programs. What we offer works and it works consistently. In fact our CASPer preparation programs have been proven to significantly increase applicants' CASPer practice scores by 23%. Our programs are in high demand and we are certain they will also work for you as well.

Why did we write this book?

In our opinion, there is so much misinformation online and offline. From online forums to university clubs and even some university guidance counselors and official test administrators. While some of these sources are well intended (not all are well-intended), the level of misinformation is astounding. For example, in our opinion, most online forums cannot be trusted because it is not clear who the authors are, what motivates them, and thus their credibility comes into question. These forums are frequently filled with fake profiles and some of those fake profiles are official university administrators and test administrators trying to control the flow of information so only their version of "facts" is distributed. To make matters worse, some of these forums offer "sponsorship opportunities" to companies, which puts them in a financial conflict of interest. Most student clubs are also to be avoided because often they also form financial relationships with companies to support their operations and as such they provide one-sided information. Additionally, most books out there are incomplete and tend to have a narrow focus on teaching you 'tricks' about CASPer without any meaningful strategy on how to ace any possible *type* of a CASPer question. They do not focus on the big picture that is essential to your success, both as an applicant and as a future practicing professional.

What is this book about?

This book is about the big picture. It is about how to develop into a mature, ethical, and knowledgeable individual, which is essential to becoming a future practicing professional. While we spend a considerable amount of time walking you through specific instructions on how to prepare for CASPer, it is important to always remain focused on the big picture.

Who is this book for and who is it NOT for?

If you are applying to any program that requires you to take the CASPer test, then this is perfect for you. Regardless of where you start, this book has something for you, provided that you are willing to put in the hard work and invest in yourself. Getting into a competitive professional school is challenging. As is being a practicing professional. In fact, the journey is very difficult and very expensive in terms of time, money, and energy. We do NOT share any quick 'tricks', 'shortcuts', or 'insider' scoops like some of the other books out there. Therefore, this book is NOT for anyone who is looking for an easy, cheap, shortcut to get in.

We do not share any such trick or shortcuts because:

A) There are no tricks or insider info that can help you, because you cannot trick your way to becoming a mature, ethical professional. Rather, you must put in long hours of self-training. Think of it this way, just like a professional athlete trains for years - on average ten years, hence the "ten-year rule" - to get to that level of proficiency, wouldn't it make sense that our future doctors, teachers, nurses and dentists, who deal with people's lives, put in the effort to learn the skills required?

B) Sharing 'tricks' or 'insider scoops' would be highly unethical and against our philosophy of what a good professional is all about and you should be immediately alarmed if a book or admissions company claims to be sharing 'insider' information.

C) We have a strict policy at BeMo to only help students who are genuinely interested to become a caring future professional and help their community, rather than those who may be primarily motivated by financial security, status, or social pressure from their parents and peers.

How should you read this book?

We recommend that you first read the book cover to cover and then come back to specific chapters for a detailed read. The more you read the book, the more you pick up the essential strategies that you may have missed. It is important to note that there is a lot of information in this book, and if you try to do everything at once, it may seem overwhelming and discouraging. Therefore, it is best that you first read this book for pleasure from cover to cover, and then take one or two points from one of the chapters and gradually start to implement our recommendations.

To your success,

Your friends at BeMo

CHAPTER I

What is CASPer?

CASPer simply stands for **C**omputer-based **A**ssessment for **S**ampling **Per**sonal characteristics. It is a web-based situational judgment test (SJT) claimed to assess how you approach and consider different real-life scenarios and the problems within them. SJTs have been used by organizations around the world for hiring employees and they represent an old technology. The CASPer test was modeled after SJTs by McMaster University for screening their medical school applicants. Since then CASPer has been licensed to a for-profit corporation to administer the test, while McMaster University remains a part shareholder of this corporation. The test is currently used as part of the admissions process by several academic programs and is no longer limited to medicine. Unlike more traditional examinations, each scenario in CASPer is either described in a stanza of text, or in the form of a video clip. The applicant is then presented with three questions pertaining to each scenario. These questions are designed to assess your ability to consider each and formulate a sound response to the challenges presented in each question. Importantly, you only have a total of 5 minutes to answer all three questions for each scenario. The entire test consists of 12 such scenarios lasting 90 minutes in total with a 15-minute optional break at the halfway point.

The rationale behind using CASPer

Now, you may also ask yourself "what is the rationale behind using CASPer?" Or, you may wonder why professional schools care so much about your personal and professional characteristics. To answer those questions, we need to start at the beginning of the story.

Although CASPer is not limited to medicine, as we mentioned earlier, it was originally created by McMaster University for their undergraduate medical training program. In 2005, a research study published in the New England Journal of Medicine, showed that the majority of complaints about physicians are related to lack of professionalism, rather than lack of scientific or clinical acumen (https://www.nejm.org /doi/ full/10.1056/ NEJMsa052596). Patients simply did not feel comfortable with the way they were treated by their physicians. This had nothing to do with the physicians' technical competencies or abilities, but rather with their demeanor and personal attributes. For example, physicians were deemed to be unsympathetic, unethical and to lack compassionate demeanor or appropriate communication skills. Thus, medical faculties were asked to put in place admissions procedures that would identify individuals who possessed those certain personal attributes and characteristics that would be essential for a medical student and a future clinician.

Around this time the Michael G. DeGroote School of Medicine or the McMaster University Medical School as it was known prior to 2003 also introduced an in-person form of SJT called the multiple mini interview (MMI) as a potentially more reliable and valid measure of candidates' personal characteristics. The commercial success of the MMI as an allegedly more reliable and valid predictive tool for assessing essential personal and professional characteristics, and the unreliability of autobiographical sketches and personal statements appears to have led McMaster to develop the CASPer test. In fact, CASPer is essentially a web-based multiple mini interview or an online situational judgment test. This is why CASPer questions are very similar to MMI questions.

In short, the creation of the CASPer test was a response to the need for more doctors who not only have an impeccable grasp of the technical aspects of their profession, but also have strong soft skills that are essential to the delivery of appropriate care and the building of a trusting patient-doctor relationship. Today, many different programs beside medicine use CASPer, because it has become a commercial entity marketed to as many programs as possible. Regardless, all programs hope to be able to assess each applicants' ethics, empathy, communication, resilience, judgement, and teamwork. Whether or not CASPer is actually able to measure these qualities and whether or not it has any impact on the level of complaints against professionals is another story and we'll get into that later, but the point is this: being a future professional is much more than just knowing certain facts and figures about the profession. As a professional you must be an expert in your area of expertise as well as make a meaningful and caring human connection with those you serve. Establishing trust through making a connection is important because if your patients, students or clients trust you, they are more likely to listen to your expert advice and adhere to your prescribed treatment. At the same time, a compassionate and ethical individual is less likely to take advantage of those under their care at a time when they are at their most vulnerable.

Do situational judgement tests *really* work?

Before we haste into specific preparation strategies we need to take a closer look at situational judgement tests because it will provide you with more depth of understanding of such tests. The more background knowledge you have, the better you can prepare for these tests because you will know the larger purpose of the test and this will help in structuring your responses.

Remember, CASPer (and its in-person twin sister, the MMI) is merely a situational judgement test or SJT. SJTs present an outdated technology, which have been around for decades, especially in the workforce for hiring new employees. SJTs work by placing applicants in hypothetical real-life scenarios and evaluating their on-the-spot behaviors. The assumption is that this methodology gives a better indication of the applicants' true behaviors.

However, in our opinion, there are multiple problems with SJTs such as CASPer (and MMI) as follows:

Problem #1:

The use of hypothetical scenarios may force applicants to provide hypothetical responses. The applicants know that the only way to do well is to provide a hypothetical response that is socially acceptable. Therefore, instead of providing what they *really* would have done, they provide what they think is going to get them accepted. This means that such tests might not be able to discern the true personality of applicants, rather at best they can detect their ability to formulate hypothetical responses to hypothetical situations.

Problem #2:

Applicants coming from a higher socioeconomic background appear to be better able to formulate a socially acceptable response because of their upbringing putting others at a disadvantage. In fact, two independent studies of medical school admissions in the United States and Canada by SortSmart showed that all admissions screening tools, including CASPer, appear to be more likely to select applicants coming from higher income families. The results for the two studies can be found in the following URLs:

American Study: https://sortsmart.io/blog/united-states-medical-school-admissions-study

Canadian Study: https://sortsmart.io/blog/canadian-medical-school-admissions-study

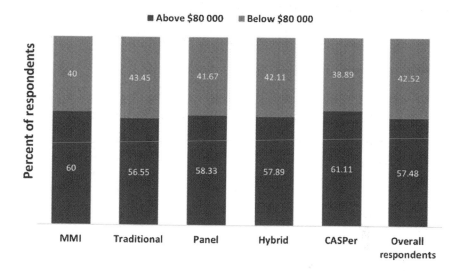

Figure 1. Showcases how the wealthy are the most represented group regardless of the admissions tool used to select them. (printed with permission from SortSmart Candidate Selection Inc.)

A survey of American medical school students and residents showed that majority of selected applicants ("overall respondents") come from high income families earning more than $80,000/year, while the median household income in the United States is ~$60,000/year according to the U.S. Census Bureau. The results further indicated that there are no significant differences between the percentage of wealthy applicants in the overall pool of respondents and the pools of respondents selected using the various admissions tools highlighted. This is similar to other published reports indicating that applicants from higher socioeconomic status appear to score higher on situational judgment tests compared to those from lower socioeconomic status and those from underrepresented minorities. (See Acad Med. 2015 Dec; 90 (12): 1667-74. doi: 10.1097 / ACM.0000000000000766.

which can be found at https://www.ncbi.nlm.nih.gov/pubmed
/26017355)

Judging whether a response to a usually very delicate or
stressful imagined scenario is appropriate can vary across cultures.
These tests are singularly guided by accepted western cultural
norms. This can pose significant challenges to non-native
applicants, new immigrants, or those who are immersed in another
culture. The diverse cultural makeup of the United States, the
United Kingdom, Australia, and Canada, for example, makes this a
significant issue for applicants. Evidently, at the 2016 medical
education conference in Canada, the New York Medical College
(NYMC) reported that underrepresented minority applicants
scored lower on CASPer, and that males scored lower than females,
indicating a possible gender bias as well.

Problem #3:

The claims that these tests are "immune to test preparation" is a
difficult one to accept. The tests aim to assess personal and
professional characteristics, qualities that any good parent or
education system aims to instill in its pupils.

Personal and professional behaviors are not inherited but
learned, claiming otherwise is irresponsible and can amount to
discrimination.

Problem #4:

SJTs have not been validated to correlate with actual on-the-job
behavior and the best correlation found to date has been self
reported by the creators of the for-profit company selling such
products. In their pilot study the company founders report a mere
low correlation of $r = 0.3–0.5$ between the computer-based SJT
and test scores in future medical licensing examinations. First, the
study seems to suffer from the law of small numbers and
confidence over doubt bias because of its small sample sizes and the
conflict of interest by the authors and the host university. Second,
note that a) the test is merely a predictor of future test

performance, not future on-the-job behavior, and b) the correlation is weak at best because a correlation factor of 0.5. Briefly, correlation factor or "r" value can range from 0 - meaning zero correlation between two variables - and 1 – meaning 100% correlation between two variables. Therefore, r value of 0.5 translates to the ability to explain 25% of the variance between the two variables. Imagine going to a doctor who claimed to be able to make a correct diagnosis only 25% of the time!

Problem #5:

SJTs are unable to measure the level of motivation of each applicant. Motivation is important because motivation directs behavior, not test scores. Furthermore, motivation is not correlated with gender, race, or socioeconomic status.

The point is this: you must question everything. All the time. Never take anything at face value, even if it comes from "official" sources. Best practices change and evolve continuously as new discoveries are made. From treatment options for illnesses to admissions practices. Progress has been driven by those who have an insatiable appetite to continuously push the status quo. Those who have an aversion to the phrase "because it has always been done that way." For example, Galileo was mocked, ridiculed, and imprisoned because he refused to believe the accepted dogma that Earth is the center of the universe because he had scientific evidence that suggested otherwise. Many years later his work was praised by Albert Einstein and Galileo eventually became to be known as the father of modern physics.

Marcus Aurelius said it best almost 2000 years ago: "Everything we hear is an opinion, not a fact. Everything we see is a perspective, not the truth."

This attitude is paramount to our future as a society. As a future professional, you have the responsibility to push the boundary of current "truths" and advance new discovery and improvement. Most discoveries are proven incorrect as new information becomes available. Therefore, by definition, everything we know now is wrong. It just happens to be what we know at present while we wait to make new discoveries.

Characteristics tested by CASPer

As indicated above, CASPer is claimed to be able to detect characteristics admired by professional programs. The test has become a screening tool for personal and professional characteristics or "non-cognitive" skills and capacities that cannot be deduced by grades and standardized test scores.

The test in essence claims to test the following in applicants:

1. The ability to make mature decisions under stress.

2. The ability to make ethical and moral choices given a challenging scenario or ethical dilemma.

3. The capacity to resolve conflicts with peers and superiors.

4. The ability to solve complex problems by considering various perspectives and points of view, while staying objective, rational, and open-minded.

5. The ability to realize team dynamics and become a valuable part of a team.

6. The capacity to fluently communicate thoughts with individuals of varying degrees of knowledge and authority.

In short, CASPer is claimed to test the soft skills or people skills of applicants. That is, those qualities and characteristics that are required to practice the "art" of any profession. Thus, it should come as no surprise that your CASPer test accounts for a large percentage of your pre-interview score and how you perform on this test will likely determine whether you will be invited for an interview.

Now that we have looked at how CASPer started, and what characteristics the test measures, the following chapter will look more in-depth into the structure and various components involved before we move onto specific preparation strategies and sample questions.

CHAPTER II

Structure & Components

H ow is the CASPer test structured?
The CASPer test is comprised of 12 scenarios: 8 video-based and 4 text-based. Each video scenario includes a short video of about 60 to 90 seconds in length. You will not be able to pause or rewind any of these videos. In fact, you are not able to pause at any point during the test. The test is meant to be written in one sitting and whether or not you type in your answers, it will continue to advance forward toward completion. The refresh and back buttons on your browsers have also been disabled and using those buttons may lead to lost time. Therefore, it is critical that you take the test on a computer that is reliable using a stable internet connection to avoid interruptions.

Following each scenario, you are presented with 3 open-ended questions. You will have a total of 5 minutes to answer all 3 questions. These real-life scenarios may or may not be related to the actual profession to which you are applying, and technical knowledge of the profession is not required. Some of the scenarios are simply personal type questions such as, "Describe a time when you had to overcome an obstacle," or "have you ever been in conflict with a superior or authority figure? How did you resolve this conflict?" The remainder of the scenarios will include cases of conflict of interest, ethical dilemmas, conflict resolution, and others. (More details about CASPer question types to follow in *Chapter VII: 21 Possible Types of CASPer Questions*).

Break time

Keep in mind that half way through the CASPer test, there will be an optional 15-minute break. This break time can be used for you to catch your breath. This would not be an ideal time to reflect on the past responses as that will only distract you and cause additional stress. Instead, what you can do is breathe, get your stress levels down and prepare for the second half of the test.

Technical issues

Since the CASPer test is administered online, technical issues can arise. For example, you may notice the computer screen freeze, the videos not loading, or you may be unable to submit your answers. If this happens, make sure you make a note and report any problems to the administrators of the test. Furthermore, CASPer raters are trained to flag instances of tech issues if they believe you were caught off mid-sentence due to technical difficulties. We will discuss how the test is scored in Chapter III.

CHAPTER III

How is CASPer Scored?

Possibly the most frequently asked question about CASPer is, "How is CASPer scored?". While this isn't a secret per se, it is not something admissions offices or the administrators will actively provide you with, although the publicly available research by CASPer creators provide many hints. Keep in mind that knowing how the scoring system works is not the same (and not even as important) as knowing what the assessors are looking for when scoring the questions. It also shouldn't change your approach to the questions or how you construct your responses. It should most definitely not change the way you think about becoming an ethical and mature practicing future professional. Below we will breakdown who will assess your CASPer test, how they are trained, and importantly how CASPer is scored.

Who scores your CASPer test?

Before we go into the grading, lets first look at who rates your CASPer response. The raters for the test are individuals from all walks of life. They include practicing professionals, professional school students and residents, members of the public, undergraduate students, or anyone provided with a registration code which allows them to go through the online training process and become a CASPer rater. The online training program provided to the potential assessors gives them an overview of the test and how it should be scored. Each rater only sees one scenario for each applicant and they are not aware of the applicant's personal identifiers. Thus, each applicant's CASPer test is claimed to be seen by 12 distinct raters. This supposedly helps to increase the inter-observer reliability of the test. The raters are given general information about the concepts important to each scenario and major ideas that should be discussed, but they are not provided with an answer key because there are multiple ways to formulate an appropriate response and similarly there are many ways to formulate an inappropriate response to complex hypothetical situations presented during the test.

How are the raters trained?

Each CASPer rater is given an online orientation and training session on the logistical aspects of marking CASPer tests and the criteria they must apply to each response when grading test responses. The raters are then provided with an online multiple-choice quiz to assess their suitability as a rater. If they fail any question, they are shown the correct answers automatically and then retested on the same quiz until they get all the questions right. This is the aspect of the test that is claimed to minimize subjective judgment in favor of objective assessment criteria - notice that we use the term "minimize", not "remove". Tests with written answers marked by humans, even ones who are experts in this field, will never be 100% objective.

Now you might be thinking "Wait, so the CASPer raters get a multiple-choice quiz and are not tested using CASPer itself?!" If this question popped in your head, you are already thinking like a true professional and we're glad you are part of the team. To answer your question, based on publicly available information CASPer raters are not tested using the CASPer itself. It is odd that the raters themselves are not chosen based on their performance on the same test, especially if the test is meant to judge personal and professional characteristics better than anything else. Wouldn't it make sense for a doctor advocating a remedy to take her own medicine?

How is CASPer scored?

CASPer responses are graded using a numerical Likert-style scale. The scale runs from 1 to 9 with 1 signifying a "unsatisfactory" response and 9 signifying a "superb" or superior one. Although all three responses to the questions for the same scenario will be graded by the same rater, the score that you receive is representative of your overall performance on that station. For instance, if during one of the scenarios you take a lot of time to provide a well-thought out and mature answer to only one of the three questions and only have limited time (or no time at all) to answer the remaining two, you can still score high on that station, granted that the answer you provided to question one was strong, appropriate, and professional. This is why it is important to focus on formulating well-thought out answers and having a strategy for CASPer (both of which will be discussed in *Chapter VI: 17 Proven Strategies to Prepare for and Ace Any CASPer Test*), rather than increasing your typing speed. Remember CASPer is not a test of your typing skills, instead claiming to test of your personal and professional skills. A mature professional recognizes what matters most and focuses on quality rather than quantity.

Flagging an Answer

Raters are not required to comment on the score they give, or provide any feedback justifying the score. However, they do have an option to flag an answer due to ethical concern, indications of unprofessionalism, or to indicate the possibility of technical glitches that may have led to a poor performance at a given station. A rater will flag an answer for the following reason as the publicly available CASPer rater training by the administrators of the test highlights:

"The response given indicates a dangerous, unethical, unprofessional or potentially harmful approach to the scenario that displays a clear deficiency in the candidate's ability to appreciate the complex ethical issues raised."

If a response is flagged, the rater is then obligated to comment on why they flagged the answer. This mechanic acts as something of a fail-safe for a candidate's application process. The flagged response and the rater's comments will then be reviewed by an admissions officer or committee. If it is judged that the rater was excessively harsh in their judgment of the response and provided the remainder of the applicant's responses scored well, this red flag can be overlooked within the context of that candidate's overall application. However, multiple red flags on an applicant's test score are likely to result in rejection of the application.

You may be asking yourself, "What happens if my test is marked by a rater with excessively high standards?" This is unlikely because importantly each scenario is claimed to be marked by a different rater making it very unlikely that you ended up with 12 raters that were all difficult graders. Furthermore, given the instruction CASPer raters receive with regards to objective marking criteria, the marking system is set up to account for the possibility that some raters have more critical approaches than others. When marking CASPer, a rater will be given a series of candidates' responses to the same scenario and questions. The advantage in doing this is two-fold: the rater can apply the same criteria to multiple applicants' responses rather than having to shift focus between subject matter every time and the applicants have a different rater marking each question rather than one continually harsh (or lenient) assessor for their whole test. This is claimed to improve fairness and give a more accurate representation of the applicants' interpersonal skills and ability to respond to the challenging scenarios CASPer presents.

Example of a Likert Scale:

1	2	3	4	5	6	7	8	9
Unsatisfactory		Good		Very Good		Excellent		Superior

As the raters analyze your responses, they will be applying the CASPer marking criteria to each answer. Application of the criteria will vary from question to question as you may be given a scenario centered around informed consent, but then be asked a question on patient autonomy.

Here is an example of a scenario medical residents might receive. Note, if you are not applying as a medical resident, you are unlikely to receive such a question, but we want you to follow along anyways as we make an important point. Later when we get to sample questions, you'll notice that most CASPer scenarios are actually not related to the field of studies but rather they relate to every day scenarios. Nevertheless, the following serves an excellent example for the point we are trying to make in this section.

Question 1:

"You are a surgical resident in an outpatient clinic seeing a patient who has been diagnosed with ovarian cancer that requires surgical intervention. You are discussing the details of the surgery and explain that both open and laparoscopic oophorectomy are possibilities in her case. How would you ensure any consent this patient provides for surgery is informed?"

Question 2:

"After your discussion, the patient expresses that she does not wish to undergo surgery, stating that she would like to give chemotherapy a chance first. How would you respond to this decision?"

First note that advance technical knowledge of "open and laparoscopic oophorectomy" is irrelevant and if you see a technical term in CASPer it is just meant to shake you up a bit to see how you manage your stress. As you can see, this sample question encompasses numerous areas and deals with several ethical concepts. While the first question specifically asks about informed consent, the second then adds a dimension of patient autonomy and could even be argued to branch into evidence-based medicine.

Bottom line, from a rater's point of view, the more dimensions of the question you can demonstrate to have recognized and considered, the better the grade you will receive. In this example, you would need to appreciate what important aspects of the patient encounter contribute to informed consent (e.g. proposed procedure, details, possible alternatives, risks and complications and consequences of doing nothing) and recognizing that - provided the patient has the capacity to make their own decisions about their healthcare - making the decision to decline surgery, although potentially inadvisable within the context of their illness, is a patient's inalienable right as part of their autonomy.

How long does it take for your school to receive your CASPer score?

The results are distributed to your preferred schools within 3 weeks of test completion.

Will you receive your CASPer score?

You will not receive your CASPer score and they will not provide you with any form of feedback. The administrators will send your CASPer scores directly to your preferred schools.

Will I have to take the CASPer test each time I apply?

Your CASPer results are valid only for one admissions cycle and you will have to re-write the test in the future if you are applying again. Therefore, it is critical that you do well the first time you apply so you'll hopefully never have to write this test again.

CHAPTER IV

Admission Statistics & Why You Must Ace CASPer

How important is your CASPer score? How is it weighted in the overall admissions score? The answer to this question differs for each school. Each school can use your CASPer score in any way they see fit to decide who is admitted and who is rejected. Some universities tell you exactly how they will use your CASPer scores while others aren't as transparent. The best way to find out is to consult the official university admissions website and contact the admissions office for the most up to date information. Regardless, your CASPer score is likely going to be a significant, if not the deciding factor between an acceptance letter and a rejection letter.

In order to appreciate the importance of CASPer, one particular University provides the best hint at how other schools may be using your CASPer score. Recall that CASPer was originally introduced by McMaster University and since then the test has become a for-profit venture and McMaster remains a part owner of this new company that administers CASPer. Given this information it may be possible to deduce that other schools that are adopting CASPer are most likely also following a similar approach to the use of CASPer scores in their overall admissions decision.

McMaster medical school receives roughly 5,000 applicants for about 200 spots. This means the success rate is a mere 4%. McMaster also indicates that CASPer accounts for a whopping one third of the pre-interview score for each applicant. Next, by looking at McMaster's official admissions statistics for previous years, you will notice two very interesting patterns. First, a lot of applicants with excellent MCAT and GPA scores do *not* gain admission. Second, roughly 30% of accepted applicants have average or below average GPA and MCAT scores compared to the average accepted scores!

Thus, regardless of how well you do on your admissions test and how high your GPA score may be, without a competitive CASPer score you will not be invited for an interview and your application will likely be rejected. On the other hand, even if you have a below average GPA and admissions test scores you can still gain admission, if and only if, you ace your CASPer test.

This general conclusion can be applied to other schools and programs that are currently utilizing the test. Again, the best way to find out is to contact the official admissions office or the official admissions statistics. You will notice that almost all schools utilizing CASPer accept students who have less than outstanding standardized tests or GPA scores. Some schools even include a strict cutoff for CASPer scores and if you don't meet the cutoff your application is automatically rejected even if you have perfect grades and standardized test scores. Therefore, you must prepare for and ace your CASPer test. There are no shortcuts and no exceptions. If you are still skeptical, ask yourself this: why would a school go into the trouble of using a test if it was not important?

CHAPTER V

Top 2 Myths about CASPer Preparation They Don't Want You to Know

Before we begin reviewing sample scenarios we must first identify the top two myths about how to best prepare for this test. We will then turn our attention to specific preparation strategies, followed by different types of questions and sample questions and answers in subsequent chapters.

Myth #1: "There are no right or wrong answers."

This is stated on official admissions and test administrator's websites. This is a complete myth and it is commonly misunderstood by students that get rejected. Notably, although there are no specific right or wrong answers when it comes to the various scenarios you encounter on the CASPer test, there are appropriate and inappropriate answers that you can provide. If this was not the case, then a lot more individuals with fantastic GPA and standardized test scores would be admitted to any university that requires CASPer, but of course we now know that is not the case. Here is another way to think about this myth. If this were true, then everyone would get accepted regardless of their performance on CASPer. The reality is this: there is certainly a difference between a well thought out, mature, professional, and articulate answer and one that is immature, unprofessional, and disorganized. It is your job to learn how to do the former and avoid the latter otherwise a rejection letter is as likely as the rising sun.

Myth #2: "You can't study for this test" or "Such tests are immune to coaching" or "You can't prepare in advance"

This is the most common and most absurd myth about CASPer. One that is again, sadly, purported by the test administrators and some official universities' admissions websites.

Our students do not require convincing because while we cannot comment about other CASPer prep programs, we know our CASPer prep programs work and the result they produce is the reason we have become the leader in CASPer preparation in the world. You are also clearly not taking such unsupported comments seriously and that's why you have purchased this book. In fact, most students also joke about this myth and comment how illogical it sounds. Furthermore, we even have scientific proof to bust this myth but before we share that with you, let's think about this myth for a moment.

What does CASPer *claim* to test? It claims to test personal and professional characteristics such as empathy, communications skills, and ethics. All these traits are *learned* behaviors. Nobody is *born* with any of these. You either learn these behaviors as a part of your upbringing or through deliberate training. Normally, but not always, people from higher socioeconomic status learn to *display* these skills while growing up because of their social environment. This is perhaps why they score better on such tests. The rest of us must learn how to display these skills actively on our own. When you understand that simple concept, you'll understand how ridiculous it is for someone to claim that it's not possible to prepare for such a test. You now have an intelligent response whenever someone says something as absurd - be they "official" sources or random online forum members, university admissions, or a malicious applicant trying to misguide others in hopes of gaining a competitive advantage. Myth busted.

If that doesn't convince you, consider this. We recently conducted a double-blind study of our CASPer prep program to examine its effectiveness. Double-blind means that neither our students nor our consultants were aware we were conducting the study until after the study completion. This is important because we wanted to avoid confounding factors that could interfere with our study. You can review the study results by visiting the following URL: https://bemoacademicconsulting.com/blog/bemo-casper-prep-and-multiple-mini-interview-mmi-prep-review-casper-and-mmi-highly-coachable

The study included 24 applicants with an upcoming CASPer test who were selected randomly to participate in the BeMo study. The applicants' baseline performance was determined by conducting a realistic mock CASPer test (CASPer SIM™) using BeMo's CASPer Prep program protocols followed by expert feedback and numeric scoring identical to the scoring system used by the CASPer test administrators. We coached the applicants by identifying areas of improvement and re-tested them using additional independent mock CASPer practice tests. Each applicant received a total of 3 practice CASPer tests followed by expert feedback.

The results speak for themselves. Our applicants significantly improved their CASPer practice scores by 23% compared to their baseline performance (and their MMI practice scores by 27% compared to their baseline performance). A 23% increase is *huge* when you are competing with thousands and sometimes even tens of thousands of applicants. Even a 1-2% increase could give you an edge in a fierce competition. 23% is the difference between a rejection letter and an acceptance letter. 23% is the difference between disappointment plus thousands of dollars in waste and enjoying a fulfilling career for the rest of your life. Myth busted again.

Effect of Expert Training on CASPer and MMI Practice Scores

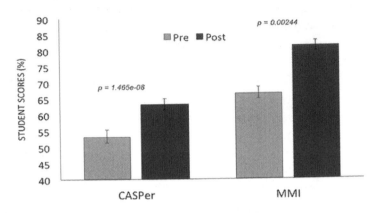

Figure 2. Applicants' CASPer practice scores improved by 23% on average after only 3 CASPer preparation sessions and expert feedback with BeMo.

The above two points are sufficient to convince the few applicants who are on the fence or mistakenly guided by the test administrators' comments. Nevertheless, the test administrators make a few other conjunctures that merit commenting here.

They say that they have done some research on their "own internal data" and that "they have not been able to find any evidence of practice effects".

It is critical to note that in their "research", they simply looked at average scores of applicants across scenarios for a given test. Then claiming that the applicants' average scores were unchanged throughout the test. For example, if applicants on average received a score of 6 out of 9 on the first scenario, they also received a 6 out of 9 on subsequent scenarios, on average.

Well, you see the flaw in this rationale? That's not practice. You don't get practice while you are writing a test. Practice happens way *before* you write the test. Furthermore, as we have always said, practice does not make perfect. Practice makes permanent. It is only *perfect* practice that makes perfect. That means you only get better on CASPer if you practice using realistic simulations followed by expert feedback so you can learn from your mistakes. How else are you supposed to get better? You will never magically learn a new skill by mindlessly engaging in the activity. Rather, you need a coach to tell you what you are doing well, and more importantly what you are doing poorly and how to do better. You keep doing this until you get better based on the judgement of an expert. Myth busted yet again.

The administrators go on to make yet another false claim. They say some companies make the claim that their preparation program is proven to increase your score but they don't know how you scored before and after your preparation. False again, we just showed you that in fact that's exactly what we did in our double-blind study (Fig. 2). We compared each of our students' baseline practice scores with their practice score following our preparation program and on average their practice score significantly increased by 23%. Bottom line, we do know how our students score in their practice tests before and after preparation and the results are clear.

But there's more. The administrators baselessly state that the performance of students taking preparation programs is likely confounded by the fact that students who use preparation programs are more affluent. Incorrect again. There is clear evidence that test preparation programs do not contribute to the well known socioeconomic bias present in professional schools. Instead studies have suggested that it is admissions screening practices themselves that are responsible for the bias against applicants from lower income levels.

Two independent studies by SortSmart in the United States and Canada demonstrated that wealth does not correlate with the likelihood of using admissions preparation services. You can view the study results by visiting the following URLs:
American Study: https://sortsmart.io/blog/united-states-medical-school-admissions-study

Canadian Study: https://sortsmart.io/blog/canadian-medical-school-admissions-study.

This makes perfect sense. The cost of our services is a fraction of what it costs to obtain a professional degree or attend an in-person multiple mini interview (in-person format of CASPer) for example, which requires applicants to travel thousands of miles and pay thousands of dollars for flight and accommodation, never mind the hefty application costs. Furthermore, professional school students on average must pay tens of thousands of dollars per year just for tuition or risk going into debt and later forced to pay all back with interest. Therefore, it's easy to see how naive and false such a conjecture appears, even without the facts that show admissions prep does not correlate with wealth.

The two studies by SortSmart, which included a random and representative sample of medical students and residents, had a margin of error of +/-5% and suggest that: admissions appears to favor the wealthy (**Fig. 3**); the wealthy are the most represented group regardless of admissions screening tool used to select them (**Fig. 4**); 94% of accepted applicants would support a new and improved admissions screening tool (**Fig. 5**); wealth does not correlate with the use of admissions preparation services (**Fig. 6**).

Admissions Favor the Wealthy

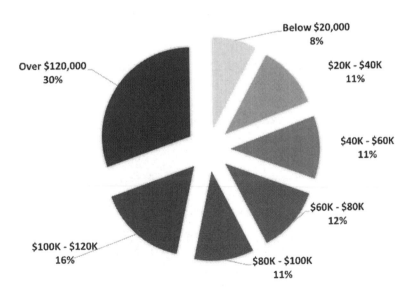

Figure 3. While the median household income in the United States is $60K/year, 69% of medical school students and residents reported household income of over $60k/year at the time of application.

Wealthy are Most Represented

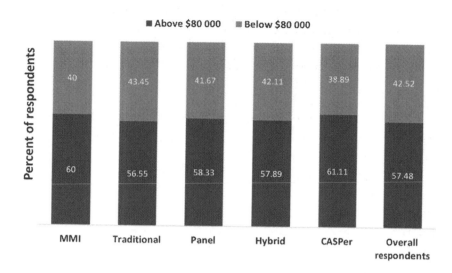

Figure 4. The wealthy are most represented group regardless of admissions tool used to select them.

Majority of Future Doctors Support a New Admissions Tool

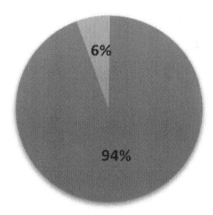

Figure 5. 94% of students and residents would support a new and improved admissions screening tool.

Admissions Prep is not Correlated with Wealth

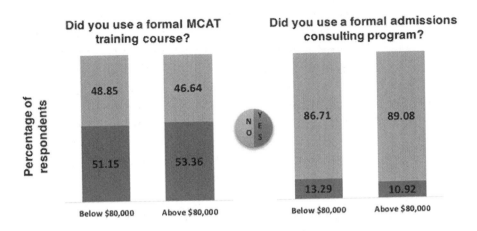

Annual household income at the time of application

Figure 6. Wealth does not correlate with the probability of use of admissions preparation services.

The findings are similar to a report by the New York Medical College (NYMC) that showed underrepresented minority applicants scored lower on CASPer, compared to other applicants, and that males scored lower than females creating a gender bias. This is corroborated by independent published studies about the Multiple Mini Interview (MMI), which is the offline version of CASPer from the same university. MMI has been found to be biased against male applicants and underrepresented minority groups score lower on these types of interviews. You can find the two studies at the following URLs:

https://www.ncbi.nlm.nih.gov/pubmed/28557950

https://www.ncbi.nlm.nih.gov/pubmed/26017355

When you thought it couldn't get any worse, the administrators go even further claiming: "We have heard students directly recommending to other students that they don't think it [preparation programs] helped them. Ultimately, it's your choice, we just don't want you to waste your money!"

Here's another false opinion spread as facts. This type of claim is vague, broad, unverifiable, and unconvincing. How many students using many different prep programs did they sample? How do they define "help"? Did it not increase their score, increase it not as much as they expected? Or did it not help with the butterflies they felt in their bellies the day of the test? Therefore, such generalizations spread as facts should be viewed with extreme caution. Second, online forum users with random names are probably not your most trustworthy options and could simply be representatives of admissions offices and administrators as discussed earlier. Third, our success rates and study results speak for themselves. The only waste of money here would be the cost to write this test plus the cost of reapplication process and loss of time if you don't prepare well in advance.

Why do the administrators make such claims? We don't know for sure. This is something you must ask them in a public forum. But here are some plausible explanations, based on our opinion.

Perhaps, they feel insecure about their test, since it has not been really validated to correlate with actual on-the-job behavior, rather barely correlates with future test performance. Maybe, that's a point of customer acquisition for them because promising to new schools that the test is better than traditional tools and "immune to preparation" might entice skeptical admissions deans. Maybe they just don't know better. Or perhaps, they simply want to defame us because they don't like the outspoken underdog and advocate of students that has been standing up to them and demanding change. We don't know and we don't care. Rather, the important question to ask is this: is this really the company that is being trusted to judge others on professionalism?

What we do know is that the for-profit test administrators do *not* offer any refunds if you get rejected. They do *not* provide any feedback. They do *not* provide you with your test scores. They do *not* have any form of satisfaction guarantee. On the other hand, BeMo does offer a bold satisfaction guarantee because we hold ourselves to a higher standard and we wouldn't create a program that we wouldn't recommend to our own friends and family, at full price. Furthermore, the reason we exist is to make sure no one is treated unfairly as a result of the current admissions practices until a fairer and scientific admissions screening process is created and adopted by most universities. In fact, a significant portion of our revenue is used for research and development of a new admissions screening tool. Regardless of what they say, we will continue to advocate for fair and scientific admissions on behalf of all students.

You now have three choices:

1. You can choose to apply to schools that do not require CASPer so you don't waste your time and money.

2. You can do absolutely nothing to prepare in advance like most students who get rejected and pretend what the "official" sources say is true because it's the easier route.

3. Or, you can reject this utterly nonsensical conjecture about preparation, stand up for yourself and get ready for your CASPer test before it's too late.

Ultimately, the choice is yours. Choose wisely.

CHAPTER VI

17 Proven Strategies to Prepare for and Ace Any CASPer Test

As previously discussed in *Chapter V: Top 2 Myths about CASPer Preparation They Don't Want You to Know,* you can and must prepare for CASPer in advance. All human behavior is learned behavior and just like any test, there are specific strategies to prepare and ace your CASPer test. Our CEO, Dr. Behrouz Moemeni, PhD was invited to write an article on the Student Doctor Network (SDN) on CASPer. The following is a combination of that original post with additional information. Note that these are the same exact strategies we use in our much sought-after CASPer preparation programs. They work and they work consistently. Therefore, take the time to read the following multiple times before you move on to the next chapter and keep referring to them as you prepare for your actual test.

Here's what to do when writing the test:

1. Read all questions twice and answer the easiest question first.

The advantages of this strategy is threefold: A) by reading each question twice you make sure you are not missing any important details and not rushing into your answers before you completely understand each question, B) answering the easiest question first ensures that you have answered at least one question before the time is up, which may still get you full marks as we discussed previously, and C) since you have read over all the questions, your subconscious mind will be busy formulating a response to the more difficult questions while you answer the easiest ones.

2. Take time to consider your answer.

In a similar way to re-reading the questions, taking a few moments to compose your thoughts and running through them in your head is a far better approach than typing down thoughts as they pop into your head. Although you won't be penalized for having a disorganized answer - provided it contains well-reasoned points - it will make the answer more difficult to read for the rater which then prevents them from giving you top marks. Don't just start typing the second you've finished reading the questions, take a moment to get your head around what's going on, then begin responding.

3. Pay attention to your spelling and grammar.

CASPer raters are specifically told NOT to penalize applicants for spelling and grammar errors. This rule was designed to ensure that applicants are not punished due to the time limit. While that rule is adhered to within the scope of its intention, it is something of an impossibility for there not to be score discrepancies between answers with no spelling or grammar errors and those that do.

It is much easier than you may think to identify those for whom English is not their first language (or generally have poor written communications skills in English), and those who speak fluent

English based on CASPer answers. More importantly, the administrators explicitly mention that CASPer is also a test of your communication skills. While significant allowances are made for answers with misspelled words or inappropriately constructed sentences, it is far less likely that you will get your point across adequately to the rater with an answer that contains either of these. Remember that the raters are human and they will subconsciously prefer appropriate spelling and grammar.

4. Read your answers over again when you are finished (if time permits).

Not only does this help with the last point by picking up spelling mistakes you may not have noticed when you were typing your answers to the questions, but it allows you to double check that you are happy with what you wrote, how it reads and how it is presented. Although you may not have time to "draft" answers to all the questions to then go back and finalize each answer, you should be able to re-read every answer before moving forward. Again, if time permits.

5. Identify the most pressing issue. ✳

Your first task is to figure out what the most pressing issue is that you are asked to address. Is someone's safety at stake or are there larger implications for the society as a whole? Generally, the most pressing issue in (almost) all CASPer scenarios is the well-being of those under your care. For example, if you are a doctor, it's the well-being of your patients. If you are a teacher, it's the well-being of your students. If you are the captain of an oil tanker, and the tanker is leaking, the most pressing issue is the well-being of your crew and the immediate and long-term impact of an oil leak on the environment. This is really important, and it comes with practice.

6. Remain non-judgmental always.

CASPer scenarios are often intentionally missing key information to see if you are going to make a hasty conclusion or if you are going to gather all the facts before making a decision. A professional always reserves judgment until after he or she has all the facts. This brings out our next tip, and I'll give you an example there.

7. Gather all the facts. Don't make any assumptions.

I just mentioned above that you must remain non-judgmental until you have gathered all the missing facts. Let's assume a CASPer scenario implies that a person is potentially intoxicated and is walking to their car in the drive away. How can you be 100% sure they are intoxicated? What if the person has diabetes and what you smell on their breath is ketoacidosis? What if they are indeed drunk, but are simply going to grab something from their car? You don't know until you gather all the facts. Importantly, if gathering facts involves having a sensitive conversation with another individual, make sure you explicitly mention it will be a *private* conversation. As a professional, you never want to have a sensitive conversion and potentially embarrass another person in front of others, unless it is absolutely unavoidable.

8. Figure out who is directly or indirectly involved.

As a future professional, you need to show that you understand that real-life situations often impact not only those directly involved in the scenario, but others who are peripherally involved as well. So let's say you are about to fire the assistant coach of your college basketball team for professional misconduct. Who is directly involved? You, the coach, and the rest of the team. Who is indirectly impacted? The college, the college basketball community at large, the coach's family, etc.

9. Learn to identify and have a strategy for each type of question.

As we mentioned earlier, it's impossible for you or I to predict what the actual questions are going to be on your real test, but if you learn to identify the different question *types* and have a strategy for each, you'll have a better chance to ace any possible question you face during the test. For example, is the question about solving an ethical dilemma or is it asking your opinion about a specific policy? Is it a case of conflict resolution or does it involve professional boundaries? We have identified 21 possible types of questions and we'll go over each of them in detail in *Chapter VII: 21 Types of CASPer Scenarios*.

10. Provide the most rational and common-sense solution that causes the least amount of harm to those involved, using simple "if, then" strategy.

A lot of times, applicants spend a considerable amount of time reading advanced medical ethics books, but that's not necessary and often leads to frustration. Remember, CASPer is meant to test your professionalism – so all you need to do is show that you can make common sense decisions and come up with rational decisions that cause as little harm to others as possible. This is best done using a simple "if, then" strategy. For example, "If after gathering all the facts I am convinced that this person is indeed intoxicated but is grabbing their phone from their car to call a taxi, then I would not interfere, but rather offer help calling a taxi for them. On the other hand, if I am convinced that they are going to drive away intoxicated, then…"

11. Don't rush. It's OK if you miss a question or two.

Unlike popular belief, CASPer is *not* a test of your typing speed. Therefore, it's okay to miss a question or two, because, as discussed earlier, CASPer raters are instructed to assign an overall score for each scenario even if you have missed a question or two.

12. If you get stuck, stick to BeMo's formula.

If you're faced with a scenario that you're unfamiliar with and are struggling to grasp, stop. Take a deep breath. Re-consider the question stem if necessary. Consider the steps we have described thus far and start from the beginning: read the question over, consider the most pressing issue, gather facts.

Don't forget, if you finish a question and feel like you did poorly or you ran out of time, remain focused and move on. One or two bad scenarios with the rest going well still gives you a great chance of scoring high. Remember, each scenario is a new set of points to score, so you can make up for low-scoring questions on subsequent ones.

Here's what to do when preparing for the test:

13. Dedicate at least 6-8 weeks to prepare for CASPer.

Since CASPer is a behavioral type test, you must start preparing well in advance because it takes a long time to develop new habits and get rid of other undesirable behaviors. In our experience it takes at least 6-8 weeks to fully prepare for CASPer.

14. Familiarize yourself with professional ethics.

Some of the CASPer scenarios discuss important concepts related to professional ethics. Therefore, it is important for you to read some general books about professional ethics. We don't recommend any specific books, but a Google or Amazon search should give you plenty of options.

15. Avoid overreliance on books and guides.

Books such as this one are a good starting point for preparing for the CASPer test, but once you have used this book to gain the essential background knowledge, it will be time to put the theory into practice, which brings us to the next point.

16. Practice using realistic CASPer practice tests.

It is understood that just like any other functional skill, the only way to improve your CASPer performance over time is by deliberately engaging in the task repeatedly. Therefore, simply reading books about CASPer or going over sample questions are generally ineffective methods of preparation on their own, unless they are coupled with practicing realistic and timed simulations. Simulations also remove the element of "fear of the unknown" and make you less nervous and more confident on the day of the exam.

17. Remember that PERFECT practice makes perfect.

Lastly, it is important to note that only perfect practice makes perfect. After all, practicing forms habits, and if you are practicing using inappropriate strategies, you are going to form bad habits, which will impede your ability to do well on this test. Using realistic simulations is great but insufficient without expert feedback. How else will you know whether your responses are full of red flags?

It is critical that you ask an expert – a mature professional, such as a practicing healthcare professional, a medical doctor, a university professor, or anyone with a higher educational background at PhD level or above – to go over your responses and give you specific feedback on your answer and how to improve. Additionally, this must not be a friend or family member so they won't hold back. This is the most effective way to prepare for CASPer. Period.

Alternatively, when you enroll in one of our CASPer prep programs, you'll get access to realistic simulation followed by expert one-on-one feedback from one of our CASPer experts who go over each of your responses, tell you exactly what you did well, what you did poorly and how to do better so you can learn from your mistakes. To learn more, visit our website at bemoacademicconsulting.com/casperprep

BeMo's Proven Formula for Acing *any* CASPer Question

Most scenarios on CASPer are based on hypothetical scenarios that describe a seemingly challenging everyday situation. Therefore, if you have a solid strategy to ace these types of questions, you are well on your way to successfully answer most of the questions on any CASPer test and if you do just that you are likely to get a higher score that most other applicants. We briefly discussed this strategy in points 5 to 8 in the previous section. Here we expand on these concepts and coalesce them into a comprehensive strategy that you can use to deconstruct and resolve even the most complex scenarios. Remember these are not CASPer skills or test skills but life skills that will help you become a better future professional and a better person.

Identify the most pressing issue.

As mentioned earlier, this is the first thing you need to learn to do. You only have 5 minutes to answer 3 questions and if you don't get this part right, you're going to give a response that may seem irrelevant or even dangerous and irresponsible. How do you do this under such time pressure? Well, firstly this will not come naturally for everyone, but it does get easier with practice. One exercise we normally do with our students in our one-on-one CASPer prep programs is to ask our students to tell us what they think is the most pressing issue after watching or reading a scenario. We keep doing this exercise with them until they can consistently identify the most pressing issue.

If you are having a problem identifying the most pressing issue, here's what to do when you watch or read a scenario: find out the consequences of doing absolutely *nothing*. For example, what would happen if someone is indeed drunk and you let them drive? What would happen if you get into a conflict with someone and you do absolutely nothing to resolve it? What would happen if one of your team members refuses to do their part and you do nothing to address that problem? Often, doing this exercise will help point you to the most important issue at hand. It will help you focus before you formulate your response. This will become clear as we go over sample questions in *Chapter VIII: Sample Question/ Expert Analysis and Responses.*

Reserve judgment until you have all the facts.

Next, you have to gather all of the facts prior to formulating a response. Remember that most CASPer scenarios have a lot of missing information. This is done intentionally to see whether you are going to assume the presence of certain facts that are not explicitly available. Mature professionals reserve judgment until they have all the facts, while being judgmental is often associated with lack of thought maturity and the ability to consider many perspectives at once.

You should not make any assumptions or hastily jump to any conclusions once you have initially read or watched a scenario. If you approach a scenario judgmentally and form a very quick and superficial decision, then you will provide a response that lacks the nuanced approach that many of these scenarios require. This is a sure way and most common way applicants get poor CASPer scores.

For example, let's say you are working in a group setting and one of the group members complains to you that some other member is not contributing as much. In such a scenario, you are missing a lot of information. What's the definition of adequate contribution? Does each group member know the expectations? Is this a one-time occurrence? Is the group member ill or dealing with other extenuating personal matters? Are the two members on good terms with each other or is there a history of animosity between the two? Clearly, you are missing a lot of information and if you jump into a conclusion and say something like "well, in this case I have no choice but to report the slacking group member to our professor" then you have already lost all points for that station because you acted judgmentally without gathering the facts first.

So how do you gather the facts since you are dealing with videos and text on your screen? Simple. You explicitly show the raters your thought pattern. Here's an example: "First, without *trs mentionner*

[making a decision,] I would have a *private* non-judgmental conversation with the two team members to gather more information." Note the emphasis on the word "private". Whenever your fact gather involves speaking to others, make sure you explicitly say that you will have a private conversation – and make this a habit in your own life. This shows that you have emotional and social intelligence and you don't want to embarrass someone by asking them sensitive questions in public. The only exception to this rule is when you have to deal with an emergency situation and you don't have the time for a private conversation.

Determine who is directly and indirectly involved

As part of your fact gathering and investigation process, you must also identify all the parties that are directly and indirectly involved in the scenario.

For example, imagine a scenario where you are the physician and you need to communicate a piece of information to a patient. Although, in the scenario there are only 2 individuals directly involved (the doctor and the patient), the delivery of the piece of information to the patient can at times, indirectly affect the patient's family, co-workers, the larger medical profession, and the doctor's colleagues. For instance, if the news is about a diagnosis regarding a terminal illness, then the information is going to impact the patient and his or her immediate family, friends and even co-workers. On the other hand, if the same news is delivered hastily without due diligence and it turns out to be a misdiagnosis, now in addition, the doctor's colleagues and the entire medical profession may be involved and impacted as a result.

Mature professionals can identify those who will be directly and indirectly impacted by their decisions. Conversely, those who do not have maturity of thought, will not be able to identify the grander implications of their decisions and will only identify those who are directly involved.

*Choose the best solution(s) based on sound rational, ethical, legal, and
scientific reasoning using "if/then"*

Once you have considered a few practical options or potential
possibilities of solutions, choose the one that is the most rational,
ethical, legal, scientifically sound decision that causes the least
amount of harm to those directly and/or indirectly involved in the
scenario. This way you can be sure you have formulated a strong
and appropriate response.

On CASPer, you will be asked to explain your thoughts and
behaviors around a specific ethical issue. You will have to share
your thought process around situations that reflect a lack of
professionalism, crossing professional boundaries and displays of
cultural incompetence.

Some of these are really complicated. So how do you make the
best decision possible, especially when they say "there are no right
or wrong answers" – which you now know is a myth?

The best way to formulate your response in a complex situation
with a lot of unknowns is by using the "if/then" strategy as you
verbalize your thought patterns for the raters.   *If →then strategy*

Sometimes, when you place your hands on the keyboard to
start writing as the clock feels like it races to 00:00, you aren't sure
what you should do. It's not clear what the right answer may be.
For CASPer, there are some contexts for which there is no perfect
answer, but you MUST report to authorities when public safety or
vulnerable individuals may be in harm's way. As long as you report
when you know you should and take the high road (which is
usually the safest road), then you won't fail the question. But, not
failing is different than excelling at CASPer.   *If stuck → report to authority*

We want to walk you through an approach that we use for
these situations when working with our students. We call it the
Punnett Square approach because it makes use of mental 2 x 2
tables, but you could also call it the "If this, then that" formula.

For example, consider the following question and again do not
get hung up that this scenario is related to medicine because it's a
very plausible scenario in any profession.

You are a surgeon. You arrive at the hospital at 7:30am to
prepare for the day. As you are changing, a fellow surgeon - a

friend of yours - enters the change room and they are acting strangely. You smell a slight scent of alcohol when they come close to you. You know that this surgeon is next in line to run the Department of Surgery at your hospital and will be making important decisions about funding and operating room (OR) time in the very near future, and you have never seen them act this way before.

What do you do?

Well at first glance you don't know if the surgeon is drunk or suffering a medical condition that gives them an alcohol breath – such as diabetes - so perhaps the answer is not as obvious, and you need to gather some facts.

Once you have had a private conversation there are two outcomes. If the surgeon is not drunk, then there's nothing to worry about as long as they are not suffering any other medical conditions that would impede their ability to perform as normal. However, this is almost impossible to deduce from a conversation and it's always best to be safe than sorry which brings us to the next possible outcome.

On the other hand, if you find out that the surgeon is indeed drunk, the right thing to do here is probably obvious to you: This surgeon should not be allowed to operate today, and their superiors should be notified that he showed up to work intoxicated. But the test isn't just about whether you have the right answer, it's about sharing how you think, your values and your personality. So, the way you break down this problem is as important as doing the ethical thing.

The Punnett Square approach breaks down your approach to thinking about this question into decisions and outcomes.

- Decision
- Best Outcome Possible
- Worst Outcome Possible

Here are some possible decisions and outcomes:

- Recommend to your friend that they do not operate today and hope they listen. Don't report the incident.

- There are no issues in the OR and the surgery goes as planned.

- The patients to be operated on today experience adverse outcomes as a result of an intoxicated surgeon. Some may even die. There is an investigation and my own license to practice is taken away for not fulfilling professional duty to protect patients from harm.

- Report the incident to your superior and the professional body that governs physician behavior in your jurisdiction. The surgeon is not allowed to operate today. They are asked to undergo a review of their recent cases to ensure there is no pattern of unsafe behavior. The surgeon gets involved with the help they need to deal with whatever led them to drink at work - a clear zone of zero tolerance for alcohol - and they return to work when ready, healthier than ever. No patients are harmed.

- The surgeon refuses to speak with me again for reporting the incident. They still somehow get the Department head job and make my life very difficult by limiting access to OR time. I have to change hospitals.

When your CASPer answer includes statements like, "If I talk to my friend to try to urge them to not operate and they don't listen to me, the best case scenario is...but the worst case scenario is..." then you're using the Punnett square to logically and clearly break down the most important issues of the question. In doing so, your decision becomes very easy to make. The answer that brings the least harm and the most benefit into the lives of patients is to report the incident. Don't forget that when you're done writing through the Punnett square, you have to write down the decision you would make so the rater does in fact know where you stand.

Obviously, when you're writing CASPer, you can't insert 2 x 2 tables into your answer. But you can think about the scenario like this so you keep clear on where you are with the answer. It will allow you to answer quickly and thoughtfully. The raters will not be left wondering if you've considered the big picture or not because you clearly have thought through the possible consequences of your actions.

Our experience is that this method prevents people from fumbling through their answers, repeating themselves and getting trapped in ethical blind spots. It also allows them to type faster and effectively. It also makes them sound professional and accessible.

Note that the things we have mentioned up to this point have to be done quickly and simultaneously in your mind as you read the scenario. However, as you initially start practicing, it is a good idea to follow the step-by-step strategy slowly and methodically in order to solidify the process. Once you are comfortable, you should be able to do this process automatically.

Master Strategy from BeMo CEO: See ethical dilemma everywhere and think like the test creators

To really get these strategies I want you to start seeing ethical dilemmas everywhere. In the ride home from school, in the grocery store, in a classroom setting, in the news, in your favorite show, even in a conversation you had with your mom this morning. Then start applying our strategies to any ethical dilemma you encounter and create a CASPer scenario and follow up questions as if you were the test administrator. You know you have truly mastered a skill when you are able to teach the material. One way to become a CASPer prep expert is to create CASPer scenarios and questions daily. Do this simple exercise for 15 minutes a day for the next 30 days and I guarantee you will notice a significant improvement. This will not only help you ace CASPer, but it will help you become a mature professional and a better person, which is the primary goal of this book.

CHAPTER VII

21 Possible Types of CASPer Questions

In the previous chapter, we showed you a proven formula you can apply to almost any CASPer question. In fact, that formula works for most CASPer questions you are going to encounter on your test. If you get good at using the BeMo formula, you are already going to do better than most applicants. But as you already know, when you are competing with tens of thousands of other applicants for a few hundred seats, you need to do way better than just above average. You need to ace CASPer and to do that, you need another set of tools: the ability to identify and have a strategy for different *types* of CASPer scenarios. It's not possible for anyone to predict what exact questions you are going to get on your test - and certainly that is not the point of this book - but if you understand that there are a finite number of *types* of scenarios, then you have a competitive advantage against almost everyone else.

We have identified 21 different types of CASPer scenarios. Almost 90% of all CASPer scenarios you are going to encounter include a combination of these different types of questions and getting 90% of questions right on CASPer is more than sufficient to get you into the accepted pool and away from the rejected pool. We could have come up with a list of 100 different types of questions but that would not be efficient, practical, or necessary for you as future professional or as it relates to your test performance. It's not even smart to aim for perfection. That's not realistic and it takes a lot more effort to move the needle from 90% to 100% than it does to go from 60% to 90%. This is something you need to learn for life which was explained in the 1800s by Vilfredo Federico Dmaso Pareto and later dubbed the Pareto Principle or the 80/20 rule. If you are interested to learn more do a quick online search for "80/20 rule" or "Pareto Principle".

Lastly, note that even though CASPer was initially intended for medical students, these 21 different types of scenarios show up in all disciplines that require CASPer.

Different types of CASPer scenarios

1. **Conflict of interest:**

    This is rather straightforward. Conflict of interest refers to any scenario where individuals, contrary to their obligation and absolute duty to act for the benefit of those they serve, may be tempted to exploit their relationship or status for their own personal benefit. This happens every time some individual or organization is unable to perform their obligations because of a competing self-serving interest. For example, a hospital director who insists on using products from a company that she receives gifts or compensation from would be said to be in a conflict of interest. A teacher who is assigned to grade test scores of his close friend's son, is also in a conflict of interest.

    Here are a few really interesting ones for you to think about. A university professor in charge of education research who creates an admissions screening for-profit company from his publicly-funded research is said to be in a conflict of interest because he would not be able to objectively judge new advances if such advances threaten the existence of his newly formed for-profit venture. A university professor who is a director of a for-profit company, such as an admissions screening company, has a conflict of interest if she appears in company related activity – for example, an information webinar for students taking the admissions test - and introduces herself as professor of the university instead of one of the directors of the company. Similarly, a public university that is tasked with advancing knowledge is said to be in a conflict of interest when its ability to advance discovery is impeded by its interests in a for-profit spin off company. Any of these sound familiar?

2. **Ethical / moral dilemma:**

Ethical dilemmas occur when an individual is faced with a scenario in which any decision taken will lead to some form of moral violation or harm to individuals involved. For example, let's say you are a doctor in an emergency room and you simultaneously receive two patients both requiring a kidney transplant to survive but you only have one kidney available. Or, you witness your best friend stealing from her abusive boss at work who has not paid your friend for the past 2 months. The test wants to see evidence that you can make ethically and morally sound decisions even when scenarios appear to be impossible.

3. **Professional boundaries, obligations, and ethics:**

These types of scenarios deal with instances in which effective and appropriate interactions and relationships between the professionals and the public are violated. For instance, a professor having relations with his student outside of the academic setting would be categorized as a violation of professional boundaries.

4. **Scope of practice**:

All professionals are said to have a certain scope of practice. These are laws and regulations that define the procedures, actions and processes that are permitted for a licensed professional. For example, only medical doctors have it within their scope of practice to prescribe medication. If any other professional prescribes medication, they are said to be acting outside of their scope of practice. Just like a physician who has specialized in the neurology cannot advise on the pathologies of the kidney. They would be acting outside of their scope. Similarly, a math teacher is best suited to teach math and not genetics.

5. **Social and current events awareness**:

Some CASPer scenarios specifically test your awareness of current events and news about the profession. Although these are rare, it is a good idea for you to be aware of all the news and challenges faced by your future profession. The best way to do that is to read the news on the websites of the organization's regulatory body.

6. **Personal questions**:

In this type of question you may be asked to, for example, describe a time when you have had to overcome a major obstacle, or describe how you would go about solving a conflict with a superior. These draw upon your past experiences and what you have learned from them. For these types of questions, you need to review your applications and do some reflective thinking and write down all the possible CASPer type scenarios you had to deal with. You also want to know what you did in each scenario and what you *learned* from the experience. It's totally O.K. if you made a mistake in the past, everyone does, what is not O.K. is if you did not learn anything. Therefore, for such scenarios make sure that you verbalize what you learned from the experience in addition to what you did. This is also the type of question that requires advance preparation because you are likely not going to come up with good examples on the spot, especially when test date anxiety kicks in full gear and you have only 5 minutes to respond.

7. **Autonomy support:**

Autonomy support refers to the right of individuals to make decisions about their own well-being without their provider trying to force their own judgments. People's autonomy to think, decide, and act freely must be respected. This is referred to as patient autonomy in medicine and it does allow the health care provider to educate and inform the patient using the latest scientific evidence so that the patients can make an informed decision. But the health care provider is not allowed to make the decision *for* the patient or force them to choose a treatment. Another example is when lawyers provide expert solutions to their clients. Lawyers can only present any possible solutions and outcomes based on their expertise but cannot make a decision on behalf of their client. The same concept is equally important in other professions and in all circumstances the professionals' job is to educate those under their care, based on their expertise in the field so that care receivers can make sound decision autonomously. You must apply this mindset in your daily life and on CASPer whenever you are perceived an expert.

There are only extreme cases when professionals can violate this rule such as when an individual is found to be not of sound mind or physically incapacitated to an extent that makes him or her unable to communicate and make decisions. In other extreme cases when someone is likely to cause harm to themselves or others, the ethical obligation to support autonomy is replaced by the ethical, and in some

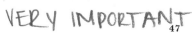

case legal, obligation to intervene and provide the best care for optimizing health. Therefore, it is important for you to keep good common sense as your best friend in life and for your CASPer test. There are always exceptions to the principles discussed and you must develop the maturity of thought to exercise good judgment and flexibility when faced with extreme cases.

8. **Informed consent:**

Another concept related to autonomy support is informed consent. Once you have provided the best possible solutions to those under your care, you have to make sure that they fully understand the solutions and their consequences by answering any and all questions so that they can make an informed decision. Once care receivers are fully informed, they can provide an informed consent to receive or refuse a specific course of action. For example, as a nurse, you must address all questions about a treatment option or request the help of a doctor to do so, when the questions are outside of your scope of practice. An excellent exercise for you to do right now is to think of at least 5 different professions and come up with examples of how autonomy support and informed consent are integral part of these professions. Then apply this to 5 different every day scenarios that involve an expert and a novice or a supervisor and a subordinate.

9. **Evidence-based practice:**

Practicing professionals are expected to make decisions and provide care and expertise based on scientific evidence rather than gut feeling or personal opinions. In the absence of scientific evidence, the best source of information is experience accumulated in the profession such as case studies. Therefore, whether you are a medical doctor, a teacher, a dentist or a speech therapist, your decisions must be based on sound evidence.

DECISIONS BASED ON EVIDENCE

Note that this is another part of your fact gathering procedure in complex problems with many unknowns and can be applied to every day scenarios. This is indeed the point. Remember that CASPer does not test your knowledge of any specific profession, that's something you learn when you get accepted. However, the test wants to find out whether you understand these concepts and can successfully apply them to your everyday life before they even consider you as future professional. Therefore, when you communicate your CASPer responses you have to take care to explicitly let the raters know that you are making a certain decision based on evidence.

10. Rural vs. city practice:

As the name implies, this requires you to be aware of the demands and challenges you would face if you were to practice in a rural setting. What are the challenges of working in a rural setting? What are the advantages? Who comes first when considering rural versus city practice, the care provider or the care receiver? Who should decide whether someone is ought to practice in the city or a rural area; the care provider? The care receiver? The government? You must know the answer to these very importantly questions and be able to provide your genuine response if such questions appear on your test.

11. Legal awareness:

This type of scenario requires you to be aware of common sense legal vs. illegal procedures. We discussed some of these items such autonomy support, informed consent, and evidence-based practice. In general, any decision you make must be legally sound in almost all circumstance. We say "almost all" because there may be cases when doing what is legal might cause more harm to those involved. These cases are rarely presented in CASPer but are most challenging because they provide a seemingly impossible ethical dilemma for the untrained test takers and generally for those who lack deep maturity of thought.

While you must always follow the rules of the law, there are times that a legal issue might be outdated and must be reformed and modified by the legal system. In fact, this is how the legal system in countries that use the "common law" system works, and the common law system is practiced by almost one third of all countries around the world including the United States, the United Kingdom, Canada, Australia and New Zealand. Laws are continuously modified to keep up with the changes in our social environment and advances in technology, science, and general human understanding.

As a disclaimer note, we are not lawyers and we cannot provide any legal advice because it is outside of our "scope of practice" – you see what we did just there? If you want to learn more you must contact a lawyer. However, note that CASPer is not a test of your deep and detailed legal awareness, rather common sense because common law is based on common sense.

12. Alternative solutions:

In almost all professions, there are alternatives to generally accepted practices. For example, in medicine, alternative solutions include those provided by homeopathic medicine, naturopathic medicine, and chiropractic medicine. In teaching, alternative to traditional schooling would be homeschooling or boarding schools. In short, these are scenarios that require you to show awareness of alternative solutions and professions and when and how, if at all, you might recommend such a solution.

13. Non-Judgmental approach:

Now, this category is a very special one, because as you recall from our BeMo formula, we talked about how you need to approach all scenarios from a non-judgmental approach so that you do not jump to any hasty conclusions or take any extreme positions. All scenarios somehow fall under this category, since you should always approach any scenario non-judgmentally and objectively.

Here's an exercise for you to see this in real time. Think about the last 2 important decisions you had to make quickly about a situation or a person. Did you gather all the facts first or did you jump to a conclusion right away? How was your action influenced by your initial rash judgment?

14. Conflict resolution:

This type of scenario, as the name implies, deals with real life scenarios that require you to intervene to resolve a conflict. This can be an internal conflict, a conflict between two individuals unknown to you, or a conflict between you and a superior, a peer, or a colleague. The scenarios will vary in detail, but the essence remains the same. You have to show that you are able to maturely and professionally resolve any conflict and come up with a mutually acceptable solution by all parties involved.

15. Global issues related to the profession:

There may be scenarios that assess your awareness of global issues that might impact your future profession. Once again, the only way to show such knowledge is to continuously read articles, scientific papers, and reports related to your profession from international governing bodies. After all, if you are truly interested in your future profession, wouldn't it make sense that you obsess over everything there's to know about it?

16. Cultural sensitivity:

As a future professional you are going to encounter people from different cultural, social, racial and religious backgrounds. Often such differences lead to different behaviors, expectations, and beliefs and your job is to show your understanding without any judgment while providing the best care and service possible. For example, what would you do if you were a teacher and a student objected to an exam date due to a religious holiday? Will you come up with a solution to make sure the student is accommodated, while being fair to other students? Or, will you retain a strict exam date?

17. Empathy:

The capacity to understand, to be sensitive to, and to experience the feelings of others, is a critical skill in any profession. When you understand those you serve, you are better able to react and attend to their needs, inquiries, and fears. Importantly, when you are truly empathetic, you can foster a trusting relationship, which in turn promotes better care delivery because when those under your care trust you they are more likely to listen to your recommendations and implement your expert solutions.

18. Collaboration:

All major discoveries and advances in human history have been due to collaboration between many individuals. In fact, there aren't any professions we can think of that don't require collaboration or are at least enhanced by cooperation amongst a group of individuals. Not surprisingly, some CASPer scenarios specifically test your willingness to cooperate with peers, colleagues, supervisors, and even individuals from across professions. For example, one of the sample scenarios on the test administrator's website shows a group team meeting by 3 students working a team-based project.

19. **Policy:**

These questions will ask for your thoughts on a newly proposed or controversial policy. Any time you are asked about your views or opinions, there are certain steps you should take in order to formulate a positive and appropriate answer. Always avoid stating your opinion or taking a side on an issue without considering all sides of the argument.

The best way to approach policy type questions is as follows:

First, begin with an introduction: this should be a general statement that shows your awareness of the policy, the complexities surrounding the issue, and why such a policy may be required in the first place. Starting with an introduction will show the interviewer you have a good grasp of the topic being discussed and that you are aware there are multiple sides to the issue. Additionally, referring to any recent news regarding the issue will demonstrate your knowledge of current events.

Once you have introduced your answer and spoken generally about the complexities, you may begin examining the specific benefits and drawbacks that need to be considered prior to formulating a decision. At this point you will provide pros and cons from the points of view of those affected by the policy. Keep in mind that you should begin with the positives and negatives from the patient, student, or client's point of view before the positives and negatives for the physician, pharmacist, veterinarian, or other professional.

After you have thoroughly presented the pros and cons to show that you have the capacity to consider multiple perspectives, you will then, based on the evidence that you have presented, discuss where you stand on the issue. A common misconception is that the most important part of your response to a policy question is the ultimate decision you make; this is not the case. Instead, what matters most is your ability to demonstrate that you can take a step back and articulate your thought process when analyzing a complex issue. When committing to a final stance on a policy issue, it is a good rule of thumb to side with the option that does the most good and least harm for those involved. Alternatively, rather than taking a side on the issue, you can provide a unique solution or compromise that would benefit all parties involved.

In general, when it comes to policy type questions, avoid taking an extreme viewpoint, providing one-sided answers, or allowing your emotions to guide your responses. Take a step back and consider the pros and cons for all individuals affected by the policy. And finally, remember that the way you approach the question and discuss your thought process is far more important than your ultimate decision. These issues are controversial for a reason: there are strong arguments to be made for both sides!

20. **Confidentiality**:

As a professional you have a moral and even legal obligation to keep all information about those under your care confidential at all time. This means you must not reveal the details of any of your conversations or findings about your care receivers to anyone who is not directly involved in providing care for them, including your own close friends and family members. You have to truly understand and display a genuine appreciation that care receivers are revealing very sensitive and sometimes embarrassing information to you as a professional. Therefore, maintaining confidentiality is critical to maintaining a trusting relationship similar to displaying a sense of empathy as we saw earlier. Just like everything else we have talked about, maintaining confidentiality is critical to your daily life.

For example, how would you feel if you found that your best friend revealed your deepest fears to complete strangers who then used it against you or made fun of you? You would probably never trust your friend with anything sensitive again and will not ask for their help in the future.

21. **Communication:**

Just because raters are asked to ignore spelling and grammar mistakes, it does not mean that you can simply type a few words hoping that the raters will be able to understand your thought pattern. In fact, this is probably the most important skill you must demonstrate, and we intentionally left it for last because it is *that* important and you will be tested on your communications skills on every single question.

How do you demonstrate excellent communications skills? First, think back to some of the tips we provided in the previous chapter. In order to communicate your reasoning, you have to take the time to read each question twice to make sure you fully understand the question and gather your thoughts before you start typing. Second, take care to explicitly explain how you would react in a given scenario because if you miss any details, the raters will interpret that as carelessness. Lastly, have a clear beginning and an end. The raters have to understand what you are trying to communicate and how you reached any conclusion.

The best way to understand these concepts is to see them in action in sample questions and answers. In the next chapter we're going to go over a full CASPer test consisting of 12 scenarios each with 3 follow up questions. As you go through these sample questions you should write a note beside each scenario indicating the type of question involved. This is a good exercise to get you to think in terms of *types* of questions rather than getting overwhelmed by an infinite number of possible questions and scenarios.

CHAPTER VIII

Sample CASPer Scenarios with Expert Answers

The following is a list of sample scenarios and follow up questions plus our expert analysis and response. To get the most out of this section, use these sample questions as a practice exam by generating your own answers, and then comparing them to the provided responses and discussion.

Each sample question consists of a stem with three associated prompts. For each prompt, we have provided two answers, one which is an example of an excellent answer and the other which would likely be red-flagged as a poor or unethical answer. Throughout these answers you will find the various components of the answer noted in brackets, which will help you to recognize the BeMo formula used for each answer. After going through examples of a good and bad answer, we will then outline the rationale behind answers, focussing on what was good and bad about each response in the discussion section.

Please note that the "GOOD" answers were *intentionally* made longer than what you would typically be able to include in a real CASPer exam, in order to give you an idea of some of the topics that could reasonably be discussed for each prompt. You do not need to write as much to get a high score and in fact you should be as concise as possible. But as your mentors we want to give you the full range of solutions in as much detail as possible to enhance your learning experience.

CASPer Scenario 1:

You are at a restaurant with your grandmother and grandfather for Sunday lunch. Your grandfather seems to be a bit confused and is acting a little strangely. Your grandmother tells you that based on some preliminary screening tests, his doctor suspects that he has dementia. Later, the conversation turns to what everyone will be doing later this afternoon, your grandmother tells you that your grandfather will be running some errands for her, including going to pick up some groceries. Your grandmother then mentions that he has had to run most of their errands lately, because she has been having trouble with more physical chores due to her sore hip and "breathing troubles". She insists, however, that he only drives around their small town, which they have lived in for 35 years, and is always careful to avoid rush hour and drive slowly.

1. What would you say to your grandparents? (*communication*)

2. Do you think it's necessary to talk to their doctor or some other authority about this situation? Why or why not? (*ethical reasoning*)

3. How do you anticipate that losing one's driver's license would impact the life of an independently living elderly individual? (*empathy*)

1. What would you say to your grandparents?

BAD: I don't think that I would say anything to them. It is their decision whether or not grandpa drives and it isn't my place to tell them what to do. **(not considering the risk to grandpa and society, lacks maturity of thought)** It is also very likely that my grandpa is capable of driving in a town where he has lived in for 35 years. **(judgmental approach, assumptions)** Lastly, if there have been no issues before, I do not presume there will be any now. **(inappropriate generalization does not address pressing issue)**

1) concerns 2) + into

GOOD: In this situation, my main concern would be the well-being of my grandparents as well as that of society at large. **(problem/values identification)** I would first want to get more information about my grandfather's diagnosis and whether he had been subsequently cleared for driving by his doctor. I would also want to know what other resources are available to my grandparents, should my grandfather lose his license. For instance, could a neighbour help them, or maybe someone else from our family? Could I consistently help out? Is public transit or food delivery an option? **(information gathering)** Once we had this conversation privately, if it turned out that my grandfather's diagnosis was mild, and he had been cleared for driving, then I would not be concerned about him driving this afternoon. However, because I am concerned his condition might worsen, I might ask them if I could help them with their errands today and if I could come to the next doctor's appointment to ask some questions about my grandpa's diagnosis and prognosis, and to be involved so I can lend them a hand or help them find other resources in the future. If his diagnosis was more severe, and he was not cleared for driving, I would be more concerned about him potentially placing himself and others at risk should he continue driving. I would express my concerns in a non-confrontational way and offer to take them to get groceries after lunch. I would also talk to them and find out what kind of resources are available to them within the community to help them get their groceries and other chores done. I might offer my services or help from another family member who I know is available, or suggest to them that for

(A) *(B)*

safety, my grandmother drives, while my grandfather goes in for groceries. **(solutions, if/then)** By talking to my grandparents, finding out the severity of the diagnosis and whether my grandfather's driving has been assessed, I would be able to ensure their safety as well as that of society in general in this situation. **(summary)**

DISCUSSION: In this scenario, the main issue is the potential risk that your grandfather could be posing to himself, as well as society, by driving. Your main aim as you work through the question is to figure out how to quantify that risk, and then work through solutions based on the various risk levels that you have identified. In the "BAD" answer, the individual appears to either not recognize the risk or does not want to get involved. Both are potentially red flags from the raters' point of view. The applicant takes a judgmental approach and assumes safety, thus neglecting potential risks. The "GOOD" answer shows someone who is willing to have an open discussion with their grandparents to ascertain the actual risk involved in the situation. They demonstrate that they have considered the potential for evolving risk in this situation by discussing how they will address the present risk, as well as the actions that they will take to mitigate risk in the future. They also demonstrate the ability to approach the problem from multiple angles, by discussing various ways in which they would try to help their grandparents to address this problem.

→ various angles to approach problem

2. Do you think it's necessary to talk to their doctor or some other authority about this situation? Why or why not? (ethical reasoning)

BAD: Yes, I would absolutely talk to their doctor about this situation. My grandfather is putting his own life and that of others at risk. **(jumping to conclusions, judgemental and possible privacy violation)** I would want to set up a meeting with his doctor and attend the meeting with my grandparents. It would be better if I am there, as I would be more competent to understand the severity of the situation and relay the information to my grandparents. **(false assumptions, sense of arrogance, red flag).**

GOOD: Whether I spoke to an authority about this situation would depend on a couple of factors. Although it would be difficult to report my grandfather for unsafe driving in this situation, it might be necessary if I believed that he was putting himself or society at large at risk. Knowing my grandparents to be kind and reasonable people, I would first have a private discussion with them about this matter, and try to determine whether his driving had been assessed and whether they had any concerns about his safety as a driver. **(information gathering)** From there, if I continue to be concerned about my grandfather's safety as a driver, I would express my safety concerns to them, at which point they would hopefully recognize the issue and we could work together to find a solution that allows them to get the things they need, without my grandfather having to drive. I suspect that this course of action would solve the problem. However, if I did have serious concerns about his driving, and my grandparents for some reason refused to stop my grandfather from driving, I would have to report him to the police or some other authority, to prevent harm from coming to society or my grandparents. **(solution)** Though this conversation would be difficult, I feel that it is something I would have to do if this was the case, for the safety of all involved. **(summary)**

necessary to REPORT if at large risk

Even if difficult → have to do it for SAFETY OF ALL

DISCUSSION: This question is assessing your ability to recognize and mitigate risk. It is also examining how you would deal with a potentially difficult conversation with your close family members. The "BAD" answer is simply too short and assumes that both your grandparents and their doctor have failed to do an adequate assessment of the situation. Further, it shows a lack of understanding and good ethical judgement by implying that the applicant would talk to the doctor without the grandfather's consent. Lastly, the applicant assumes his grandparents are not competent to understand the potential risks, which is both judgemental and disrespectful. In contrast, in the "GOOD" answer, the applicant starts off by identifying safety as their principal concern in this situation. They then go on to acknowledge the difficulty of this situation, as well as the necessity of ensuring that everyone is safe, making them come across as sensitive yet motivated to do the right thing. They do not jump to conclusions about their grandparents or their doctor, and instead seek to clarify the situation by asking their grandparents more questions. They provide a couple of solutions, based on the perceived risk level, and clearly indicate under which circumstances they would feel obligated to report their grandfather.

3. How do you anticipate that losing one's driver's license would impact the life of an independently living elderly individual? (empathy)

BAD: Elderly people really shouldn't have a say in losing their license, especially in the context of the potential harm they could do to society because they tend to be bad drivers who cause accidents. **(judgemental)** Once, I saw an elderly lady run directly into a motorcycle while making a left turn. When I stopped to see if she needed help, she accused the bike of running into her and explained that she was on her way to the casino. Clearly, she was confused, and her license should have been revoked long ago by her doctor. **(possibly dangerous, not realizing that she could have been confused due to a medical condition)** The situation taught me that old people like her are unsafe drivers and a hazard to those around them. **(generalization, stereotyping, red flag)** After this experience, I would have a very low threshold for revoking the license of an elderly person. **(future application, red flag)**

GOOD: Losing one's driver's license can be very difficult for anyone and even more so for elderly individuals, especially those who live in rural or remote areas and have limited access to public transport because it would limit their sense of autonomy. **(empathy, summary)** For both sets of my grandparents, who live in small towns and don't have access to public transit, it would make it almost impossible for them to access basic things like food, money, and medical care. For my paternal grandfather who lives on a country line outside of rural area, who is the primary caregiver for my grandmother who has dementia, a loss of license would prevent him from caring for his wife and engaging in the social activities that bring him joy, like going to church, volunteering, and exercising. Taxis are expensive and hard to afford for elderly individuals like my grandparents, who didn't expect to live well into their 80s or 90s, leaving elderly individuals in rural areas dependent on rides from family or friends. **(personal example)** Thus, losing one's license could have a large detrimental effect on the overall physical and mental well-being of an elderly person. **(what I learned)** Knowing this, as someone who hopes to work with elderly individuals someday, I think that it is very important to recognize the activities that are important to them and find ways to help them to continue to do those activities while promoting a sense of autonomy, even when unable to drive. **(relating to future)**

DISCUSSION: This is a personal question exploring the applicant's ability to empathize with others. In the "BAD" answer, the personal question format is followed, however the applicant's tendency to paint all elderly people with the same brush following a single bad experience is concerning. Further, her account of the incident inadvertently reveals that her overly judgemental behavior may have prevented her from considering that the accident she witnessed may have been caused by an acute medical condition, such as a stroke. Her reaction to the incident as well as their summary of what she learned and how she would apply it to the future demonstrates a lack of empathy and a tendency to generalize, both of which are red flags. Conversely, the "GOOD" answer shows a strong positive regard for the elderly, as the applicant uses their personal experience with their grandfather to illustrate the important points. The applicant clearly has a capacity for empathy and understands the multiple ways in which a loss of license can negatively impact elderly individuals. The concluding sentence suggests a thoughtful approach to the elderly, one which respects their need for autonomy, thus protecting their health as much as possible, while ensuring the safety of society.

CASPer Scenario 2:

You are the coach of a woman's softball team. You recently told your players that they could vote for a captain from among their peers. Two girls were nominated. The first candidate is popular with her teammates; however, you have noticed that she tends to belittle new and less experienced players. She is also known as a bit of an irresponsible partier, and you are concerned about the negative influence she may have on the team as a leader. The other candidate is quieter, however seems more organized and is kind and welcoming to new team members. You count up the ballots and realize the first candidate has won.

1. As a coach you have the power to veto the team vote, would you exercise that authority in this scenario? Why or why not? (*ethical dilemma*)

2. If you did overturn the team's decision, what would you say to the first candidate if she came to your office demanding an explanation? (*conflict resolution*)

3. How would you describe your leadership style? (*personal question*)

1. As a coach you have the power to veto the team vote, would you exercise that authority in this scenario? Why or why not?

BAD: As a coach, I would have to do what's best for the team, and in this case, it is inappropriate to have a woman who is known as a drinker and partier as well as a bully in a leadership position. Thus, I would choose the other woman as captain. **(jumps to conclusions without gathering information or thoroughly considering the implications of their actions on the team)** I think as the coach I know what is best for the team and therefore should have the last say. **(lacks a collaborative approach and effective decision-making skills)**

GOOD: Though I have the power to veto the team vote as the coach, there are a number of factors I would have to take into consideration before doing so, most important of which would be the impact of this matter on the overall cohesiveness and subsequent performance of my team as well as the psychological well-being of both women. **(non-judgemental, problem**

identification) Before making a decision, I would want to sit down with both women to talk with them privately, starting with the woman who had won by team vote. **(private conversations)** During this conversation, I would want to assess both of the women's readiness for taking on a leadership position. Particularly, for the woman who has won, I would want to find out whether she values inclusivity and recognizes the negative role that excessive alcohol consumption has on performance, if she does indeed engage in such activity. **(non-judgemental approach, information gathering)** Because team cohesiveness may be negatively impacted if I go back on my word after telling them they could choose a captain, if she expresses understanding and a willingness to work on her behavior and lead the team in a way that is in line with these values, then I would give her the captain position. I would also talk to the second woman, and if she was interested, offer her a secondary leadership position based on her strengths. Alternatively, if the woman selected by the team was less willing to recognize how her behavior impacts team dynamic, then I might instead decide to talk to both girls and have two captains, assigning both duties according to their individual strengths. If the selected woman was completely unwilling to change her ways and, based on my assessment during our conversation, likely to be disruptive or even corrosive to the team dynamic, then I would be forced to make a unilateral decision as coach and appoint the other woman, despite the potential risk of losing the team's trust and alienating the player, because I would be concerned that having a player like this in a leadership position could be detrimental to team performance and cohesion. Ultimately, I will continue to monitor and assess the performance of whoever ends up becoming the captain and will be ready to find a replacement if they are found not to be fit for the role. **(solutions, if/then)** In summary, in this scenario, discussing the situation with the two individuals, gathering their insight and assessing their readiness for leadership positions would enable me to make the best decision for my team, while treating both women and other team members fairly. **(summary)**

DISCUSSION: It is clear from the stem that, as a coach, you are concerned about the potentially negative impact that the selected *think about big PICTURE*

team captain could have on the overall team dynamic. However, this must be weighed against the negative impact that going back on your word may have, as well as the potentially detrimental effect that your decision could have on the candidates themselves. As a coach, your priorities are the well-being of your players as well as the overall performance of the team, both of which are influenced by team dynamic, as well as the team's trust in you, as a coach. Though it might seem that the simplest solution is to appoint your preferred candidate, as seen in the "BAD" answer, this course of action could potentially alienate one of the candidates and negatively impact the overall team dynamic. To avoid this, it is important that you remain non-judgemental, and avoid jumping to conclusions about the selected candidate. The best way to achieve this is to take the time to sit down and talk to both candidates, assess their readiness for leadership and then work out a solution with them, based on these discussions.

2. If you did overturn the team's decision, what would you say to the first candidate if she came to your office demanding an explanation?

BAD: I would probably just tell her that she lost fair and square. **(lying, red flag)** She really shouldn't be upset about this outcome anyway, because drinking and partying are inappropriate behaviors and, really what did she expect, she clearly isn't an appropriate candidate! **(judgemental)** It is also likely that people just voted for her because she is the popular choice. Besides, if she wants to continue to play for me, then she'll have to do as I say. **(non-empathetic, not considering potential implications on individual and team)**

GOOD: If I overturned the team's decision and made the announcement without discussing it with this player first, she would be understandably upset, and this is not something I would do without first discussing my decision with her. My main concern in the situation would be addressing my player's feelings and making sure she continues to feel welcome on the team, as well as minimizing any potential for this to negatively impact the dynamic of our team. **(problem identification, empathy)** After inviting her into my office to discuss the issue privately, I would commend her for her bravery in approaching me with these concerns, because my not telling her about the decision prior to announcing it to the team was a hurtful thing for me to do. I would then apologize to her for having handled it in this way. After this, I would try to get her perspective on the issue and figure out what she was hoping to accomplish by discussing the issue with me. **(information gathering)** If, based on our discussion, she is upset about the loss of a leadership opportunity, I would have a frank, but kind, discussion with her about our team values, and work with her to find an alternative leadership opportunity on the team that would allow her to further develop her skills so that she may be a better candidate for next year. If, on the other hand, she has come because she is feeling hurt, betrayed, or angry with me for choosing another player over her (and is maybe even considering leaving the team), I would be honest with her about why the decision was made, while re-enforcing her unique strengths and the important contributions she makes and value she provides as a member of our team, even in a non-leadership role. **(solution, if/then)** By having an honest, but kind, discussion with her, and apologizing for the way I handled the situation and made her feel, I would hope to be able to rebuild trust with this player and retain her on our team. **(Summary)**

DISCUSSION: This question assesses how you would utilize your interpersonal problem-solving skills to deal with the upset player. Again, as the coach, your priority is the well-being of your players as well as the overall performance of the team. Your answer should include a consideration of how your actions may have impacted this player as well as what you will do so that the both of you, and the team as a whole, can move past this incident and return to working productively together. In the "GOOD" answer, the applicant demonstrates empathy for the player, by recognizing and acknowledging how their own actions might have made the player feel. They then work with the player, focusing on the individual's strengths, to re-build trust and re-engage the individual with the team in a different role. Through their answer, this candidate has demonstrated empathy as well as strong leadership and team building skills. The "BAD" answer does quite the opposite; the "coach" shows a distinct lack of empathy and emotional intelligence by lying to the player, which is a red flag, and generally refusing to take responsibility for their actions.

3. How would you describe your leadership style?

BAD: I am naturally a very strong leader. **(vague, arrogant, not addressing the question)** I am good at identifying problems within my team and then coming up with solutions to address them. I always focus on doing what is right for the team and using my strong teamwork and communication skills to inspire them to be their best version of themselves. **(needs examples to demonstrate this implicitly rather than stating explicitly)** I believe that in order to be a leader, you need three things: a strong vision, a great team, and strong communication skills. My role model for leadership is Steve Jobs, because of his highly innovative and visionary thinking. **(not well integrated, and not addressing the question)**

GOOD: When in a leadership role, I have often been described as "a quiet leader, who leads by example". **(summary/interpretation)** I believe this is due to my tendency to spend more time listening then I do talking, and my belief in setting a good example for my teammates. As the captain of my rugby team, this strategy helped me to bridge the gap that had formed between two factions of our team, the forwards, and the backs, who blamed each other for recent losses. This "gap" caused a literal gap in our field coverage, with the backs blaming the forwards for being out of shape and the forwards blaming the backs for having weak contact skills. **(the problem)** Acknowledging that I couldn't see the whole field and gathering perspectives from both sides, I was able to identify the crux of the weakness in our team, which was a lack of on field communication and understanding between the two sides which led to neither side being able to support the other in play. I brought it up to our coach and suggested that we have the players

personal questions → include example

switch positions occasionally in practice, so that both sides would learn how the other side's plays worked and would thus be better able to predict where they would be and provide support. Further, I recognized that as fly-half (coordinator of the backs) I needed to work out a way to better communicate our plays to the forwards and vice versa. Together, the scrumhalf (coordinator of the forwards) and I devised a system facilitating on field communication between the two factions and decided to set an example by connecting with both sides more regularly. **(intervention)** As a result of these efforts, the two factions dissolved, and our team won the next couple of games and made the play-offs for the first time in over 5 years. **(result)** The experience taught me the value of listening and perspective gathering in team-based problem solving. **(lesson)** As a future leader, I will continue to put my listening skills to work, gathering relevant information from my team, before implementing changes. As someone who believes that actions often speak louder than words, especially when setting team culture, I will always strive to be a leader in change by implementing changes to my own behaviors first. **(future application)**

[handwritten: What you learn]

[handwritten: ACTIONS>WORDS]

DISCUSSION: In this case, the "GOOD" answer makes use of an interesting narrative to answer this personal question. Not only is this answer more memorable, because it includes a story, but it also clearly outlines a problem, how the individual solved it using their leadership skills, what they learned from the situation and how it will apply to future situations where they are called on to act as a leader. Contrast this to the "BAD" example, where the candidate explicitly states that they are a strong leader without providing any specific examples of their leadership skills, which sounds arrogant. This brief and disorganized answer really makes it difficult for the reader to assess whether the candidate is a strong leader.

CASPer Scenario 3:

Your best friend, Kate, recently lost her beloved dog, Lucy. Kate feels she is finally ready to get another pet and has been looking at adopting a new furry friend. The adoption agency requires a fully fenced yard, however Kate lives in an apartment building. This wasn't a problem with Lucy, as Kate loved to take her for lots of long walks and was able to exercise her off-leash at a nearby dog park. The adoption agency, however, has a strict policy against adopting out their animals to people without fully fenced backyards, and requires photo evidence of a fenced yard. Kate asks you if she can use photos of your backyard to include in her application package.

1. What would you do in this situation? (*ethical dilemma*)

2. Do you think that pet adoption agencies should have such strict policies surrounding who they will and will not allow to adopt a pet? Why or why not? (*policy*)

3. Describe a situation when you had to say no to a friend's request for help. (*personal*)

1. What would you do in this situation?

BAD: I would tell Kate that it was unacceptable for her to be asking me to lie on her behalf, even if her dog did just die. **(judgemental, unempathetic)** A true friend wouldn't put their friend in this kind of position, and, as a supposedly reasonable adult, she should be aware of the legal ramifications of acting in a fraudulent manner. **(more judgemental, self-centred)** If we got caught, she could get the both of us in trouble, which just isn't worth it to me just for her to be able to adopt a dog. **(unempathetic)**

GOOD: In this situation, though I do want to help my friend with something that is important to her, I would not want to do so by helping her lie to the adoption agency about her backyard. **(problem identification/values)** I would start by talking to my friend, emphasizing that I want to help her in any way possible. (**non-judgemental, private conversation**) I would try to further clarify the specific requirements of the adoption agency and how strict they are in terms of their backyard requirements. For instance, would they be satisfied with a home visit and meeting Kate in-person instead? I would also suggest that we call the adoption agency, or visit in person, to discuss the issue with them. (**information gathering**) If they were amenable to doing a home visit or their requirements weren't as strict, then I would help Kate with the rest of the adoption process. If this didn't work, and the adoption agency was firm in their requirement for a fenced backyard, then I would maybe suggest to Kate that she look for a new pet at another agency, with less strict requirements. She could also consider a private pet adoption or choosing to move to a house with a fenced yard. If Kate refused all of these solutions, and still insisted that I provide her with photos of my backyard, I would have to refuse, as I wouldn't want to be involved in lying to the adoption agency. (**solutions, if/then**) Thus, by clarifying the true requirements and working with Kate to find an alternative solution, I would be able to avoid lying to the adoption agency, while still helping Kate to find a new dog.

DISCUSSION: This question is looking at the applicant's ability to navigate the legal and ethical issues presented in the stem while still helping their friend. Essentially the key to this stem is to remain non-judgemental, and find an alternative way of helping your friend, that doesn't involve lying or otherwise doing something unethical. The "BAD" answer does a good job of recognizing the legal and ethical issues presented in the stem but doesn't address the emotional needs of Kate and provides a response without any information gathering. The answer comes off as judgemental and blaming, as the author righteously berates Kate for even asking them to be involved. This demonstrates a lack of willingness to help others as well as a lack of empathy. In the "GOOD" answer, the applicant sticks to their guns, by refusing to do anything fraudulent, *but* still comes across as caring and empathetic, by trying to help Kate in other ways. This applicant gathers information about the situation from Kate and the shelter, before proceeding to present various ways in which they could still help Kate, based on her needs and the limitations imposed by the shelter. This applicant comes across as moral, caring and emotionally intelligent.

2. Do you think that pet adoption agencies should have such strict policies surrounding who they will and will not allow to adopt a pet? Why or why not?

BAD: I don't think that adoption agencies should have such strict policies around adopting dogs. **(jumping to conclusions without considering alternatives)** These types of strict policies likely exclude a lot of potentially good owners from getting pets, which just isn't fair. Further, with so many animals in shelters, they really can't afford to be overly selective about who they are giving them too. If these animals don't get adopted, the unfortunate truth is that they will be destroyed. In my opinion, destroying the animal just because there weren't enough potential adopters with fenced yards is a crime. Further, not having a fenced yard may force the owner to interact with their dog more, because they have to take them out on walks several times a day. Overall, I think that pet shelters should not have such strict policies because it harms both the pets and potential owners. **(only presents one side of the argument, not showing consideration of all aspects of the problem)**

GOOD: There are several pros and cons to having strict adoption policies. **(summary, non-judgemental)** Having stricter policies are associated with several advantages. For instance, by having strict policies around housing and yard type, agencies can ensure that all of their dogs are going to have access to a specific environment that promotes their health and well-being. Further, someone who has selected a place to live with a dog in mind (i.e.: with a fenced yard) clearly is interested in investing in the pet for the long term. Having policies around geography can also help the shelter to maintain contact with the new owners and check in with them periodically. **(pros)** On the other hand, strict policies may not be necessary in every case and may exclude some individuals who would otherwise be loving and wonderful pet owners. Some dogs, such as toy breeds, may not require a large fenced yard, or an owner who lives in an apartment may be happy to take their dog on long walks every day. Having overly strict policies around housing type or geography may cause overcrowding in shelters, forcing shelters to humanely euthanize more dogs. On the balance, I believe that having overly strict policies may end up limiting the adoption pool and causing more harm to the shelter and their animals than good. Instead, shelters may want to consider looking at adoptions on a case by case basis, using screening tools to match pet and owner needs and technology to check in with new pet owners on a regular basis. **(provided alternative solutions)**

when asking "opinion"

DISCUSSION: This is a policy question asking for the applicant's *↓* opinion on strict adoption policies. The "BAD" answer immediately *state* states an opinion, which sets a judgemental tone for the rest of the *BOTH* paragraph. It also only considers one side of the issue and fails to *sides* consider all aspects of the problem or come up with a viable *+* alternative solution. In contrast, the "GOOD" answer shows a *pros &* thorough consideration of the pros and cons of having strict *cons of* adoption policies. It then presents a viable alternative that is in line *each* with the values presented throughout the question stem.

3. Describe a situation when you had to say no to a friend's request for help.

BAD: I recently had to say no to a friend who was asking me to help them study for a Statistics exam. Though I had helped him with the midterm and the exam for the previous semester by giving him my old course notes and coaching him through some of the problems, I had my own exams to study for, and didn't really want to continue to help him to study, because I found he really didn't want to focus during our sessions and was wasting a lot of my time. When I told him that I couldn't help him to study for the exam, he really freaked out, accusing me of being a bad friend for abandoning him when he needed me most. He hasn't talked to me since, but I feel that I did nothing wrong in this situation and can't believe he treated me that way. **(lack of empathy)**

GOOD: I recently had to say no to a friend who was asking me for help with his business, because I was feeling overwhelmed with the number of commitments I already had going on. **(addressing prompt, introducing situation)** Though it was difficult for me to feel as if I was disappointing him, I felt that I had too much on my plate to be able to help him in the way that he needed, and I was also a little worried that being involved in business together may impact our friendship. Luckily, I knew of a colleague who was looking for work, and so when I told my friend that I didn't think I could accept his offer, I was able to refer him to someone else who I was confident would do great work. He ended up calling that person and giving them the contract. He was really happy with her work and has hired her for multiple projects since. **(positive outcome)** So, though I did feel bad about saying no, it was ultimately a good decision, in terms of my own mental health, and, by looking at what my friend really needed, I was able to find an alternative solution that still helped him solve the problem (and also benefited one of my colleagues). **(what I learned)** In the future, I will continue to recognize my own limitations and to acknowledge that reaching them doesn't mean I can no longer help people, it may just mean I have to help them in a different way. **(future application)** Recognize limitations ⇒ solution for the future + what you learned

DISCUSSION: This is a personal question asking the candidate to explore a time that they had to let down a friend. The key to answering personal questions is to use a personal narrative that fits the prompt, and then describe what you learned and how you will apply that lesson in the future. The "BAD" example uses a personal narrative but fails to describe what they learned and how they will apply it in the future. Further, the narrative may not be an appropriate one to use. The candidate still clearly has a lot of unresolved feelings about the situation, which gives an overall negative tone to the story. To avoid this, try to choose narratives that have a positive outcome, or frame it positively by discussing what you learned from the situation. The "GOOD" answer does a good job of this. It describes a time they had to say no to a friend, and why this was difficult for them, but then spends more time focussing on the good that came out of it and what they learned from the experience. This answer communicates that this person values helping others but also has a good understanding of their own limits.

CASPer Scenario 4:

Stan, your university housemate, has recently decided to adopt a vegan diet. This means he does not consume any animal products, including meat, fish, milk, eggs and honey. He has become passionate about being vegan, and loves talking about how he is reducing his carbon footprint, as well as his risk of chronic disease and his contribution to animal cruelty. You and your other housemates have been very supportive so far, even trying some vegan food, which was surprisingly tasty. However, at your latest dinner Stan stated that he doesn't feel right about living in a house where animal products are regularly bought and used. He feels so strongly about this that he offers to do all the grocery shopping and cooking for everyone in the house, if you will all agree to no longer bring animal products into the house. Otherwise, he feels he will have to move out.

1. What are some of the pros and cons of Stan's offer? (*policy*)

2. What would you say to Stan and your other housemates? (*conflict resolution*)

3. What is your approach to working with someone whose beliefs are vastly different from your own? (*personal*)

1. What are some of the pros and cons of Stan's offer?

BAD: There are several benefits as well as drawbacks associated with Stan's offer. **(non-judgemental introduction)** The main benefit would be that Stan wouldn't have to move out and the rent can stay the same. **(motivated by self-serving interests)** The main drawback would be that we would all have to eat vegan. **(brief and poorly thought out pros and cons)**

GOOD: There are several benefits as well as drawbacks associated with Stan's offer. **(non-judgemental, intro)** There are several benefits to agreeing to Stan's offer. Firstly, that Stan, who is our friend, won't feel he has to move out to find an environment where he feels comfortable. **(sensitive, empathetic)** Secondly, having all of our grocery shopping and cooking done for us would be convenient and would save us a lot of time. Finally, there are all the benefits that Stan listed to being vegan: reduced carbon footprint, reduced risk of chronic disease, decreased contribution to animal cruelty. **(pros)** However, there are also a few potential cons to this situation. For instance, there may be someone else in our house who has personal or religious beliefs or even a food allergy or other health conditions that may exclude them from eating a vegan diet. Though well-balanced vegan diets are safe, I might worry about Stan's knowledge of nutrition and his ability to balance all of our diets sufficiently. Finally, I might worry that this is a lot of work for Stan to take on, and that some of our housemates may have trouble sticking to it, which may cause even more friction, if it's something they don't really believe in. **(cons)** As an alternative, I would suggest that Stan allow us to work out a plan that works for everyone. After a discussion with everyone, I believe we would be able to come up with a solution that addresses Stan's concerns while making sure everyone else is heard as well. For example, perhaps Stan can cook for anyone who is interested while respecting that if someone has some form of dietary restrictions or personal preference, should have a choice to prepare his or her own meal, similar to the choice provided to Stan. **(alternative solution)**

DISCUSSION: This question is asking the applicant to weigh the offer based on the pros and cons, thus considering all sides. The "BAD" answer only contains one pro (which is motivated by self-interests) and one con, and thus does not give the issue enough consideration. The "GOOD" answer contains several pros and several cons and outlines the possible impact it might have on all of the individuals involved, as well as society. Further, it offers an alternative solution, showing the raters that even a seemingly impossible scenario has alternative solutions.

2. What would you say to Stan and your other housemates?

BAD: I don't think that it's fair for Stan to be trying to force his views on the entire house, even if we enjoy vegan food occasionally. **(judgemental)** He should be happy that we are supportive of his lifestyle at all. I would inform Stan, and the group, that I wouldn't be participating. I would try to make him see that it's wrong for him to try and force his views onto us. He'll have a difficult time finding other housemates with an attitude like that, so I think it'd be an important thing to bring up. **(not listening to Stan's point of view, or that of the other housemates)** It'd be unfortunate if the end result of this was that he had to leave our house, but if he's not willing to change his view, then perhaps he might have to go live with other vegans. **(narrow perspective, offered one solution, judgemental tone, unempathetic)**

GOOD: I would want to talk to Stan about this privately, to learn more about his perspective and make sure he knows that I care about whether he moves out, before bringing it up with the whole house. **(private conversation)** I would start off by re-iterating to Stan how much we enjoy having him as a house mate and respect his dedication to his diet and recognizing its importance to him. **(non-judgemental, empathy)** Though I don't want Stan to move out, I also don't think it's fair for him to try to force his views on our entire house. **(values/problems)** I would then try to figure out what is upsetting him the most about living in our house. Is it just our consumption of animal products or is there another issue at hand? I would also want to know a bit more about his plan: does he anticipate any trouble balancing this with school and his other commitments? How would he feel if people continued to eat meat outside of the house? Does he feel he knows enough about vegan nutrition to make sure we're all healthy? Has he spoken to a nutritionist? Would he be happy with the house committing to a less drastic change, say eating vegan 3 days a week? **(information gathering)** If during our conversation, I discover that his problem with living with meat eaters is a simple fix (for instance, he doesn't like meat touching his food in the fridge) or an interpersonal issue with another housemate, then I might suggest we bring this up with the rest of the house, or that individual, and try to take steps to solve this problem before making any drastic changes. If Stan is adamant about the house being vegan, I would then suggest calling a house meeting to figure out how our other housemates feel. If at that meeting, the other housemates are open to the idea and Stan feels that he has the knowledge and the time to cook for everyone, then I would suggest trying his plan, maybe on a trial basis for a month or a semester, to see how it goes and then re-assess. More likely, however, that our housemates will not be interested in having a fully vegan house. In this situation, I might try to see if a compromise is possible, for instance having a vegan dinner together a couple times a month or agreeing not to buy certain products. If it is not possible to find a compromise, then Stan may have to move out. **(solutions, if/then)**

DISCUSSION: The key to answering this question is approaching it as a scenario question. The "BAD" answer is judgemental and does not provide a thorough consideration of Stan's point of view. Because the applicant immediately jumps to conclusions, they are only able to provide one possible solution to the scenario. In the "GOOD" answer, the applicant opts to talk to Stan privately before calling a house meeting. They come across as empathetic to Stan, as well as the rest of the house. By not immediately rejecting the idea, and instead listening to Stan's point of view, they may be able to help find a solution that prevents Stan from moving out, while keeping the rest of the housemates happy. By listening to all of the housemates and determining their needs, this candidate demonstrates both emotional intelligence and empathy, and would presumably be able to find an amicable resolution to this situation.

3. What is your approach to working with someone whose beliefs are vastly different from your own?

(handwritten annotation above: "always narrative")

BAD: There are a couple of steps I take when working with someone whose beliefs are vastly different from my own. After learning that we disagree on how something should be done, the first thing I typically do is to thoroughly research both of our point of views. I try to gather evidence for both sides to empirically determine who is right. Once I have determined who is correct, I bring my findings back to the other person, presenting them with my research. If they are logical, they will agree with what I have found, and then we can move past our difference in beliefs. In the future, I will continue to use this strategy to ensure that those I work with always take the correct course of action. **(no narrative, no indication of what was learned, lack of empathy and problem-solving skills)**

GOOD: When working with someone whose beliefs are vastly different from my own, I believe that the most important thing is to remain non-judgmental. **(recap)** For instance, while in university, I used volunteer with an organization that enabled me to work with local youth from low socioeconomic backgrounds, teaching them nutrition, health, and hygiene. **(role and who I worked with)** Before my first session, I had this kind of formal presentation planned, followed by an interactive game and a meal that we would all prepare together. When I got there however, I was met by a bunch of grade 9 and 10 students, running around the community center, and talking to each other in loud voices. I think that in my first 30 seconds watching them I heard about 10 homophobic or racist slurs. **(problem)** I knew the kids were joking around, but for me, this language was unacceptable. **(difference in beliefs)** However, because I was just meeting them and needed to gain their trust and get them engaged, I didn't think it was a good idea to introduce myself by immediately disciplining them. Instead, I took an extra couple of minutes and reworked my lesson plan. Since they clearly needed to blow off some steam, I put the interactive games first, the meal in the middle and decided to leave my formal presentation until after, if we had time. Over dinner, as we all sat around a big table, I decided to bring up some of the language I had heard before, asking the students what they thought the words meant. (non-judgemental) They were a little hesitant at first, but then I got some very unexpected answers; the kids just really had no idea what these words actually meant or the history behind them. So, I told them what the words meant to me, and how some of these words could be very hurtful to others, and how using these words might make others perceive them. (solution) The kids showed interest in the discussion by asking me about the meanings of a whole slew of inappropriate words. We didn't get to my formal lesson but the next time I came back, there were far fewer homophobic and racist words, and the time after that, there were none. (positive outcome) The situation really taught me to not judge people on first appearances, if I had, I would have immediately dismissed these students as a bunch of homophobic racists and missed the opportunity to teach them about the impact that their language was having on others. (what I learned) This will allow me to work more closely and effectively with individuals whose beliefs are different from my own in the future. (future application)

DISCUSSION: This question is asking the applicant to describe a time they worked with someone whose beliefs were vastly different from their own. This should be answered as a personal question and everyone has their own unique story. For example, you may want to talk about a difference of opinions in a group reach project or a time when you disagreed with a supervisor or a peer. The "BAD" response fails to use a narrative to answer the prompt. This results in a very non-specific answer that gives little insight into the applicant's experiences and skills. The "GOOD" answer provides a personal narrative about an experience the applicant had while volunteering. The applicant has chosen a narrative that answers the question and concluded with a summary of what they learned from the situation and how this will inform their future behaviour. This answer is much more memorable while providing valuable insight to the candidate's character and experiences.

CASPer Scenario 5:

You've been working at a financial consulting firm for the last year. For most of your projects, you are paired with Ryan, and the two of you have become pretty close. One Friday afternoon, your boss, Stacey, tells the two of you that she is angling for a big deal, and needs a detailed industry report on her desk by Monday morning. After Stacey leaves, you tell Ryan you are going to pick up some dinner and ask him if he would like some food or coffee. He says yes, and after a brief pause he adds "I'm totally wiped, I was going to get my guy to drop off some Adderall, the drug that's used as a stimulant to treat ADHD, to get us through the weekend, it really helps me get things done faster, do you want a couple?"

1. How would you respond to Ryan's question? (*ethical dilemma*)

2. Would you report Ryan to someone, why or why not? (*ethical dilemma*)

3. Adderall is helpful in the treatment of ADHD but is also frequently used by non-ADHD university and college students trying to improve their academic performance. Do you think colleges and universities should be more proactive in preventing widespread Adderall use among their student bodies? (*policy*)

1. How would you respond to Ryan's question?

BAD: In this scenario, I would have a couple of concerns. Namely, Ryan's physical and mental well-being as well as the physical risks that I would be taking by using street drugs. (**problem identification/ethical issues, missing legal issues**) To address this situation, I would start off by finding out why Ryan is using Adderall. Does he have a condition that necessitates it, or is this something he believes will allow him to work more effectively? Does he have a prescription? (**information gathering, non-judgmental**) If during the course of my questioning, it turns out that this is a prescription medication that Ryan uses to treat a legitimate condition, and he is simply having it dropped off by the pharmacy so that he can take his regularly scheduled dose over the course of the weekend, then I would have no concern, but I would decline his offer. If he is taking the drug as a performance enhancer because he feels unable to deal with the quantity of work we have been assigned, I would offer to recruit other team members to help with the project and maybe even suggest that he takes the night off, which might help to decrease his stress levels and perceived need for the drug. **(solutions, doesn't specify when/if authorities would be involved)** Thus, by gathering information about intended purpose of the drug, as well as the nature of our project, I would be able to protect the physical and mental well-being of my co-worker. **(summary)**

missing legal issues

GOOD: In this scenario, I would have a couple of concerns. Namely, Ryan's physical and mental well-being as well as the physical and legal risks that I would be taking by using street drugs. **(pressing issue)** My other concern would be getting the project done in a timely manner, as well as the reputation of our workplace. **(problem identification/ethical issues)** To address this situation, I would start off by finding out why Ryan is using Adderall. Does he have a condition that necessitates it, or is this something he believes will allow him to work more effectively? Does he have a prescription? The other thing I would want to know are the logistical details associated with our project, things like how long it will take us, how difficult it will be to complete and whether there is anyone else who can help us with this task. **(information gathering, non-judgmental)** If during my questioning, it turns out that this is a prescription medication that Ryan uses to treat a legitimate condition, and he is simply having it dropped off by the pharmacy so that he can take his regularly scheduled dose over the course of the weekend, then I would not be concerned but I would decline his offer. I would also make sure he is aware of the risks associated with diverting his prescribed medications and ensure he will not offer it to another co-worker again. On the other hand, if this is a medication that he is obtaining through illegal means and that has not been prescribed to him, or if it has been prescribed, but he is taking too much, I will have to decline his offer and inform him of the legal and physical risks he is taking by using the drug inappropriately. If he is taking the drug as a performance enhancer because he feels unable to deal with the quantity of work we have been assigned, I would offer to recruit other team members to help with the project and maybe even suggest that he takes the night off, which might help to decrease his stress levels and perceived need for the drug. If, despite my efforts, he insists on ordering an illegal substance to be dropped off at our workplace, I would be forced to notify our employer and the authorities of the situation. **(solutions, if/then)** Thus, by gathering information about the legality and intended purpose of the drug, as well as the nature of our project, I would be able to protect the physical and mental well-being of my co-worker as well as the reputation of the corporation, while making sure we complete the project on time. **(summary)**

DISCUSSION: Though the "BAD" answer shows good overall consideration of the co-workers well-being, it lacks consideration of the legal ramifications of the inappropriate use of prescription medications or the impact that this could have on the business as a whole or the team's ability to complete the project in a timely manner. Thus, the "BAD" answer's lens is too narrow, only considering one of the potential issues at hand. The "GOOD" answer considers all of the relevant issues, prioritizing the health of the co-worker, but also recognizing that there are other parties who could be harmed by his actions, from the main character and other workers, to the corporation. It also recognizes the inherent illegality of drug diversion. Though both answers engage in information gathering, the "GOOD" answer does so more extensively, considering some items important for helping them to get the project done. The solutions offered by both answers are reasonable, however the "BAD" answer is not broad enough in the solutions offered. In the "BAD" response, one is left unsure of when the individual would involve management or contact the authorities, if at all. The "GOOD" answer goes through the solutions, in order of the least severe scenario to the most severe, and clearly indicates when the authorities or management would be involved. The reasoning seems sound and in line with the values identified at the beginning of the stem.

2. Would you report Ryan to someone, why or why not?

BAD: I don't think I would report Ryan because it would negatively impact our friendship and our working relationship and prevent us from getting the project done in time for our boss. Sometimes it's more important to be political rather than being right. **(not considering broader implications, missing the most pressing issue)** Further, Adderall is a commonly used medication, without serious side effects, so even if he does take it, it's unlikely anything bad will happen. **(incorrect assumptions about drug safety, ref flag due to endorsement of harmful behavior)** That being said, I wouldn't want him offering the drug to other team members, because it might reflect poorly on our team or the corporation, so I'd have a discussion with him to make sure he wasn't sharing it with anyone else. Provided he agreed to this, I see no reason to report him, because it would just get the both of us in trouble and prevent us from completing the project in a timely manner. **(potential red flag for incorrect value identification or apparent lack of awareness of risks)**

GOOD: There are a couple of things I would have to consider before deciding whether to report Ryan. **(introduction, addressing question)** As an employee, my primary concerns are Ryan's safety as well as that of the other employees. **(identifying the most pressing issue)** I would also be concerned about the legal ramifications if Ryan is indeed distributing prescription drugs to other employees, our ability to get the project done in a timely manner and what would happen to the overall reputation of the company if widespread prescription drug abuse was uncovered. I would have a private conversation with Ryan to try to ascertain the reason he is using the medication, as well as whether he has a legitimate prescription. **(information gathering, non-judgemental approach)** I would also want to know if he is using more than he has been prescribed, which could pose a risk to his health and how often he offers it to other employees, which could pose a risk to theirs. I would also want to get a sense of his understanding of the potential for both physical and legal harm associated with diverting this drug. My main threshold for reporting to the authorities would be him offering the drug to other employees, because this would potentially put the health of these individuals at risk, as well as the reputation of the corporation. If, after our conversation, it seems that he has not offered the drug to anyone except for me, then I would want to know whether he has a prescription and how much he is using. If he has a prescription, is using the drug appropriately for a legitimate medical reason, and understands the risk associated with diverting the drug and can assure me he will never do it again, then I might not report him based solely on this one incident, assuming it truly is an isolated incident and out of character for Ryan. If I am at all unsure, I might ask that he talks to our supervisor about it, to make sure it never happens again. If he doesn't have a prescription, or does, but is taking more than prescribed, I would be concerned about his health and would thus report this to our supervisor or someone who can get him some help. I would also want to talk to him to figure out why he feels the need to use the medication, and whether any of these are environmental factors that we could address within our workplace to prevent these kinds of incidents from happening in the future. On the other hand, if he has offered the drug to multiple individuals and/or doesn't seem to understand the implications of his actions, then I would have to disclose the incident to our boss and the authorities, as he has been putting the health of himself and others, as well as the reputation of the company, at risk. **(if/then, solutions)** By talking to Ryan and determining the details surrounding his personal drug use as well as how often he is offering it to others, I hope to be able to prevent Ryan from having a major health complication related to the misuse of prescription medications and to prevent the potential harm that could come to other employees and the corporation. **(future application)**

DISCUSSION: Though the "BAD" answer acknowledges a consideration for the applicant's friendship with Ryan and identifies the importance of meeting work obligations, it lacks a consideration of the safety issues inherent to this stem. This answer completely lacks consideration of the negative impact that the medication could have on Ryan, if it is being misused, as well as the employees around him and the corporation. Because the values are not clearly defined, and arguably inappropriate, the solutions are lacking in depth and breadth, and it seems that this applicant is either incapable of identifying the potential risk or that their preferred course of action would be to avoid conflict, both of which are suboptimal ways of dealing with the problem at hand. The "GOOD" answer clearly identifies the applicant's values in dealing with the problem and then goes through the information they would need to obtain in order to deal with the problem effectively. The applicant engages with a non-judgemental and private conversation with Ryan, and doesn't jump to conclusions about him abusing the drug, but also outline the steps they would take to protect both Ryan and their other team members from harm if it turned out that this was a scenario in which drug abuse could be an issue. The applicant looks at the issue through a broader lens and considers the implications that this scenario could have for Ryan, themselves and everyone surrounding them. The solutions are clear and well thought out and it is easy to tell that this individual understands both the health and legal implications of this scenario and when and how they would decide to involve an authority in this case.

3. Adderall is helpful in the treatment of ADHD, but is also frequently used by non-ADHD university and college students trying to improve their academic performance. Do you think colleges and universities should be more pro-active in preventing widespread Adderall use among their students?

BAD: I think that schools should absolutely be more proactive in preventing Adderall use among their students. **(taking an extreme stance without considering the pros and cons)** Students who use Adderall, and don't have a legitimate medical condition, are using drugs to enhance their performance, which constitutes cheating. **(judgemental approach)** As such, it should be dealt with similarly to other forms of academic dishonesty, such as plagiarism. If schools choose not to take this issue seriously, they are essentially condoning cheating. Further, it's unfair to the students who are honest and don't want to use the medication, as they may receive lower grades as a result. Not punishing people who abuse these drugs may even result in more students taking them, because it will create the perception that they need them just to keep up. In conclusion, I believe schools need to be stricter about their cheating policies to prevent Adderall abuse. **(only addresses plagiarism issue)**

GOOD: There are several pros and cons to implementing more stringent policies to prevent widespread Adderall use among students. **(summary)** Though many students believe that Adderall improves their performance, studies have shown that Adderall makes no difference in exam performance for individuals without ADHD. What researchers found it does do, however, is create a sense of euphoria and the perception of improved performance in its users. This effect is problematic in terms of the potential for addiction and dependence upon stimulant medications. **(demonstration of knowledge on the topic, note this knowledge is not required and is used for demonstration only)** Thus, having more stringent policies against the use of these types of medications could help to protect students from becoming addicted to these substances, and subsequently spending a lot of money or participating in illegal behaviors to procure them. In addition, having more stringent policies and reducing student use could reduce the frequency of adverse outcomes associated with Adderall abuse, such as cardiac arrest, thus protecting student health. It will also reduce the overall demand which will lead to less illegal distribution. **(pros)** The downsides of creating more stringent policies, especially bans or punishments, drug use may include the alienation students who use it for legitimate medical reasons and the demonization of students who use it for performance enhancement. It also restricts students' right to autonomy. Both groups may thus become less likely to seek help when needed. Further, such policies may be difficult or costly to enforce; for instance, screening students before exams and searching dorm rooms randomly for illegal substances would be both cumbersome and a potential violation of the student's right to privacy. **(cons)** In conclusion, in order to protect the health of their students, universities should be more proactive in terms of preventing substance abuse among their student body, but their efforts should largely be educational, rather than punitive, to avoid alienating students who use the drugs and may need help or violating the student's right to privacy. **(solution)**

DISCUSSION: This prompt is a policy question, examining whether schools should make more of an effort to prevent Adderall abuse by students. There are a couple of different factors at play here, firstly the idea that Adderall enhances performance and secondly the risk of negative health outcomes associated with drug abuse. The "BAD" answer shows what not to do when addressing a policy question. The applicant immediately jumps to conclusions on the topic without considering both sides. Further, the applicant doesn't address the potential for harm to the students taking the drug without a prescription. As a result, the answer comes across as judgemental and one sided. The "GOOD" answer provides a thoughtful discussion of the pros and cons of having stricter policies against Adderall abuse. The answer also uses background knowledge, citing a study, to inform the answer. The applicant's consideration of how schools might try to monitor drug use is thoughtful and shows consideration of the issue from all angles. The solution provided is in line with what was identified to be the principal concern about the situation (i.e.: student health) and provides a logical conclusion to the discussion.

Casper Scenario 6:

You are a member of a study group with five of your friends. One of your friends has gotten a copy of last year's exam from one of the teaching assistants. The other students taking the course do not have access to the exams from previous years. He immediately forwards it to everyone in your group, stating that he wants to make sure you all do well. Shortly thereafter, you receive a second private email from Marcine. Marcine is a friend who you invited to the group but who doesn't hang around much with the other group members. She tells you to not open the email, because she will be reporting this breach to the professor, along with the names of the students who received the test. She suspects that the consequences will be dire for these students. She also requests that you don't warn the other group members, so that they don't have time to "hide the evidence".

1. Do you think Marcine's approach to this problem is "fair" why or why not? (*personal values*)

2. What would you do? (*ethical dilemma*)

3. In an environment where technology exponentially increases the ease with which students can access past course material, including assignments and exams, what can schools do to encourage academic integrity in students? (*policy*)

1. Do you think Marcine's approach to this problem is "fair" why or why not?

BAD: Based on Marcine's request that I not tell anyone in this scenario, it seems like Marcine is purposely trying to implicate our group members in cheating. **(jumping to conclusions)** Though I agree with her that cheating is wrong, I don't think that her approach is at all fair. I think that Marcine needs to mind her own business, and let other students deal with the consequences. **(unethical, red flag)**

GOOD: Marcine's approach to the problem is in some ways "fair", in that she is reporting students who may have an unfair advantage over their classmates for the upcoming exam, thus ensuring fairness to the students not involved in this situation. **(considering one perspective, ways in which it is fair)** That being said, she has treated the other members of the group unfairly, because she has only given me a warning about looking at the exam, and she is assuming that everyone else in the group has looked at it. She may actually be reporting students who wouldn't have looked at or used

Dont assume that students are doing the WRONG THING

the exam, even if they did receive it, which doesn't seem very fair. **(considering the second perspective, ways in which it isn't fair)** However, she could know something about the other students that I don't or there may be another underlying issue that I am not aware of. Despite this, I feel that she could handle the situation more fairly by bringing her concerns forward to the whole group and giving them all the option to delete the email. Furthermore, it is not possible to tell whether or not this year's exam is going to be the same as last year's and whether or not the TA is going to be sending a copy of last year's exam to everyone else. More importantly, it is not clear whether the TA was authorized by the course instructor or not. Therefore, I believe a decision should only be made once all the information has been discovered. **(alternative solution that would be fairer)**

DISCUSSION: This prompt presents a difficult scenario, because some aspects of Marcine's behavior are fair, whereas others are not. In the "BAD" answer, the applicant does address the issue of cheating, but jumps immediately into their opinion, making them come across as judgemental. The applicant also makes the assumption that Marcine is deliberately trying to sabotage the other group members, which may or may not be true in this case. The "GOOD" answer focusses on ways in which Marcine's solution is both fair and unfair. It admits that the applicant may not be aware of everything at play in the situation but offers a logical solution that would make the scenario fair both to the group members and the other students taking the class.

2. What would you do?

BAD: I would tell everyone else in the group what Marcine was doing, so that they too could decide whether or not to delete the email. **(no consideration of alternative options or information gathering)** I don't think that what Marcine is doing is fair, and I am concerned that she is in fact trying to sabotage the other students. **(judgemental)** This is a serious accusation that could negatively impact their transcripts and result in a serious flag on their academic records. Hopefully by telling my friends about Marcine's plans, I could get them to all agree not to use the material and prevent them from suffering any academic hardships over this incident. **(no consideration for the rest of the class)**

GOOD: My main concerns in this scenario would be the well-being of the group members, including Marcine, and maintaining fairness to the rest of the class by preventing cheating. **(identifying the most pressing issue)** I am concerned that if she proceeds to report everyone, she may inadvertently implicate some of our group members who hadn't engaged in cheating. This could negatively impact their transcript and their future. I would start off by talking to Marcine and finding out if there was any information about the situation I was missing, for instance whether she knows for a fact that everyone else in the group has already looked at the exam; whether this year's exam is going to be the same as last years; whether the TA was authorized by the course instructor; and whether or not the TA is going to be sending last year's exam to everyone else as well. I would then try to ascertain why she told only me or if she did in fact tell everyone else. **(information gathering)** If she had told everyone else, then I would maybe suggest that we also call a group meeting to make sure that everyone understands the ramifications of opening the email. If she hadn't told everyone else, I would try to convince her to do so, and if she refused, I would tell her I was calling a group meeting to inform them, because I believe that to be the fairest thing to do. If at the group meeting, everyone agrees not to use the test, then I don't think it would be necessary to report the incident. If some individuals admitted to already having looked at the exam, I think the best thing to do would be to ask them to schedule a meeting with the prof to disclose what happened. Though it would be difficult to ask my friends to turn themselves in, I think that this would be the course of action that would best preserve fairness for the rest of the class, and hopefully, the professor would recognize that they were trying to take responsibility and thus be more lenient with them. **(solution)** Furthermore, it is possible that the professor had authorized the TA to distribute the exam to everyone, in which case there would be no cause for concern. By talking to Marcine and the other group members and then deciding what to do based on whether the exam had actually been used, I believe we could come to a resolution that is fair to the rest of the class while having a minimal impact on the futures of our group members. **(future application/summary)**

DISCUSSION: There are a couple of things to consider in this scenario question: first, fairness to the rest of the class and second, the potentially long lasting negative impact that reporting could have on the individuals involved. For your group members, this could result in a flag on their academic record that could prevent their admission into other programs and securing employment. Thus, before reporting, you want to be sure of the facts and each individual's involvement. In the "BAD" answer, the applicant wants to protect their friends. Unfortunately, they don't give due consideration to the rest of the class or Marcine. Further, it is likely that simply deleting the emails will be an ineffective strategy. The "GOOD" answer shows that fairness and doing the right thing is this applicant's top priority. Fair consideration is also given to everyone in the group's feelings and futures, including Marcine. In this instance, Marcine is given a chance to redeem herself with the group, by being involved in the discussion, and the group members are given a chance to redeem themselves by either agreeing not to use the material, or opting to take responsibility and turn themselves in. In this way, the "GOOD" answer preserves fairness to the class while attempting to minimize harm to the individuals involved.

3. In an environment where technology exponentially increases the ease with which students can access past course material, including assignments and exams, what can schools do to encourage academic integrity in students?

BAD: Cheating has a negative impact on the students who engage in it, their classmates as well as the school and society at large. Because cheating can significantly impact grades, and grades have a big influence on professional school admissions, students may face significant pressure to cheat. To discourage this, schools must take a strong stance against all forms of academic dishonesty and punish any student caught cheating. Severe punishments for those caught cheating will discourage students from engaging in this behaviour and encourage academic integrity. **(extreme stance, only one solution considered)**

GOOD: There are a variety of interventions that could help schools to decrease the likelihood and frequency of cheating. Cheating has the potential to negatively impact students, their classmates and society at large. For instance, the students who cheat are depriving themselves of valuable learning experiences, while the honest students may get significantly lower grades while working harder. Academic cheating can negatively impact society as well, because grades are an important factor in candidate selection for professional schools. **(why this issue is important)** Rampant cheating may result in the selection of individuals with a worrisome pattern of unprofessional behaviors. There are a variety of ways schools could address this problem. Because technology is constantly changing, and schools are typically much slower than students to adjust, the best thing they can do is to promote a culture of academic integrity by educating students, so that even when students see the opportunity to cheat, they will refuse to take it. Schools should also research factors leading to cheating. Does the majority of cheating occur in specific programs? Why are students cheating? Is it due to heavy emphasis on grades for admissions to professional programs? If yes, has such an emphasis been supported by scientific research to show a positive correlation between grades and future on-the-job behavior? They can then put resources in place to combat these problems. Simple interventions, like asking students to leave all electronics at home during exams and having randomized seating assignments can also be effective. Finally, schools should demonstrate that cheating will not be tolerated, by seeking out cheaters and disciplining or rehabilitating them as appropriate.

DISCUSSION: This question looks at the applicant's problem-solving skills by encouraging them to delve a bit deeper into the reasons why students cheat and how we can prevent this kind of behavior from happening. To create a good answer, an applicant must demonstrate a thorough consideration of the factors that lead to cheating as well as what can be done to address them. The "BAD" answer fails to do this, by only considering one way of preventing cheating at the undergraduate level. The answer may also be interpreted as a bit too punitive and extreme. The "GOOD" answer explains why cheating is bad both for individuals and society at large and discusses a variety of interventions that schools could implement to address it. This answer shows thorough consideration of the issue.

CASPer Scenario 7:

Surveys show that though 86% of the population knows that too much salt is bad for their health, only 53% of them consider salt content while making food choices. In the UK, a public health approach has been developed to reduce the consumption of salt by the general population. Their plan involves setting a maximum allowable salt content for common foods and then engaging corporations to voluntarily commit to reducing the salt content of their products in a graduated fashion. As a result of this initiative, the population's salt consumption has decreased by 15% over the last decade.

1. What do you think is the significance of the statistic presented in the first sentence, that though 86% of people know that excess salt consumption is bad for their health, only 53% of them actually consider salt content when making food choices? (*personal, critical thinking*)

2. In countries where the provision of health care services is subsidized by the government, do you think that governments should be able to limit access to substances known to cause chronic disease? Why or why not? (*policy*)

3. Processed meat has been found to be a carcinogen in humans, putting it in the same class as smoking cigarettes. As a public health official, what steps would you take when

considering a ban on processed meats in your community? (*ethical dilemma, policy*)

1. What do you think is the significance of the statistic presented in the first sentence of the stem, that though 86% of people know that excess salt consumption is bad for their health, only 53% of them consider salt content when making food choices?

BAD: The statistic presented alludes to the fact that individual knowledge does not always inform observed behavior. **(interpretation)** So, even though individuals may understand how salt negatively impacts their health, they don't care enough about their health to modify their food choices. **(judgemental)** A similar pattern occurs with other food choices, for instance, individuals know that sugary and fatty foods are not healthy for them but continue to eat them anyways. Individuals are lazy and unwilling to change. **(red flag)** Unfortunately, this behavior pattern often results in obesity, diabetes, hypertension, and other chronic diseases. **(narrow minded)** It is very sad that these individuals do not care enough about their health to change their behavior. Thus, it is unlikely that any amount of educational intervention will address this problem. **(negative, judgemental, pessimistic)**

GOOD: The statistic presented in the first sentence of the stem alludes to the fact that individual knowledge does not always inform observed behavior. **(interpretation)** From my experience doing public health research, I know that the statistic alone does not give a complete picture of the various factors that may be influencing individuals as they make food choices. **(relating to personal experience)** For instance, our data showed that the degree to which individual behavior is influenced by knowledge is correlated to the perceived severity and immediacy of the negative effect. More importantly, through our research my group found that knowledge is not the only factor that influences behavior; environmental, cultural, and psychological needs may actually be more important in terms of influencing behavior than individual knowledge. For example, one of the diabetic patients who I

MEM patient,
valeurs, croyances → modific habitudes

interviewed, a recent immigrant from India, had trouble controlling her sugar intake (or levels) despite repeated large group educational sessions. The problem? The educational sessions focussed on choosing items like whole grains, but using traditional North American examples, like breads and pasta. Despite having a good understanding of the recommendations, she was unsure how to implement them in the context of her diet, which consisted of rice, curries, and chapatti. Providing her with ways to make her typical diet healthier eventually allowed her to get her sugars under control. **(relating to specific narrative)** This experience taught me that though education is an important piece of the puzzle, it is by no means the only piece, and if the education you are providing doesn't fit into the context of the individual's life, based on their sociocultural and/or economic context, then it is unlikely it will be successfully implemented. **(what I learned, future application)**

DISCUSSION: The question is asking the applicant to interpret the statistic provided. This question may be answered either as a personal question, or one may choose to use the discussion to showcase their knowledge of the topic. The "BAD" answer is very judgemental and assumes that the observed discrepancy between individual knowledge and behavior occurs due to laziness on the part of the individual. Assuming that individuals with chronic diseases such as obesity, hypertension and diabetes are lazy is a huge red flag. This suggests that the individual is lacking in empathy and has little knowledge of factors influencing the development of chronic disease. The "GOOD" answer uses a personal example to illustrate how and why mismatches in knowledge and behaviour may occur. This applicant provides their insightful answer by concluding with what they learned from the situation and how they will apply it in the future.

2. In countries where the provision of health care services is subsidized by the government, do you think that governments should be able to prevent access to substances known to cause chronic disease? Why or why not?

BAD: I think the government should make the ultimate decision for this if it is paying for the bills. The government always has the resources and expertise and they know what's best for the public better than anyone else. This way we can also make sure that money is not wasted because government is always more efficient with spending tax payer funds. I think the best thing is to have government to simply ban all such substances and punish people for their use and distribution to deter others. **(extreme stance, no pros and cons, judgemental, narrow minded)**

GOOD: There are several advantages and disadvantages to governments being able to prevent individuals within their society from accessing substances known to cause chronic disease in countries where healthcare is publicly funded. **(summary)** Advantages of limiting access to substances known to cause chronic disease include the reduction in chronic disease burden, thus increasing the quality of life of individuals while decreasing overall health care spending. Preventing access to these detrimental substances reduces dependence on individual change and could represent a quick and easy way to effect positive health changes within a society. **(pros)** Arguments against limiting access to potentially harmful substances could include the subsequent limitation of individual freedom of choice. In addition, adopting such a hard stance on the use of particular substances may prevent individuals from engaging in behaviors or using substances that are culturally significant to them, such as indigenous peoples of the Americas who participate in traditional tobacco smoking, thus marginalizing these individuals. Further, prohibiting access to certain substances may lead to the creation of alternative, informal markets for the limited substance or item, resulting in dysregulation and potential for contamination of the substances and more harm. **(cons)** Instead of outright prohibition of access to harmful substances, governments may consider "limiting" access to harmful substances by adding additional taxes or making them only available for sale from regulated centres. Educating the public on the dangers of using the substances, and labelling of the substances to inform consumers of the danger, such as we have seen in the tobacco industry, would also be helpful in this scenario.

97

As seen from the successful efforts with the tobacco industry, these types of efforts reduce population use of the substance and chronic disease burden, while minimizing the marginalization of specific populations and the prevention of help seeking behavior. **(providing alternative solution)**

DISCUSSION: This is a policy type question. The best way to answer such questions is to indicate the pros and cons followed by an alternative solution that maximizes the pros and minimizes the cons. The "BAD" answer does not consider the pros and cons and is hasty to act in an extreme fashion without deep thought. The "GOOD" answer, however, does a great job of demonstrating a clear understanding of some of the advantages versus disadvantages of such a policy followed by an alternative solution that works better than the proposed policy in the question.

3. Processed meat has been found to be a carcinogen in humans, putting it in the same class as smoking cigarettes. As a public health official, what steps would you take when considering a ban on processed meats in your community?

BAD: I would first find out why this substance hasn't been banned already if it is as bad as smoking cigarettes! Then after doing some research I would create a policy to make sure no company or individual is allowed to make processed meat or risk penalties such as hefty fines and imprisonment. **(extreme, lacks maturity of thought, lacks consideration of pros and cons)**

GOOD: As a public health official, the health of my community would be my main priority in this scenario, though I would also want to respect individual right to autonomy as well as the cost limitations of my department. **(ethical priorities, pressing issue)** First of all, I would want to know more about the research presented: who conducted it, did they have industry biases, has it been repeated and most importantly, what was the magnitude of the effect? Next, if I determined that the research was sound, and the magnitude of risk was large enough to warrant an intervention,

I would do a study to collect information from my community. I would want to know how much processed meat my community is consuming, how often and what the cancer rate for cancers associated with processed meat consumption is at baseline. I would also want to look at their perceptions around processed meat consumption and knowledge of the risks. **(information gathering, not jumping to conclusions, considers unique characteristics of this population)** If the consumption and baseline risk is relatively low, an intervention may not be warranted. If on the other hand, consumption and baseline risk were high, then I would proceed with an intervention. Even if the substance was found to be a significant health risk, it is unlikely that I would implement a full ban on the product, as this would constitute a violation of individual choice. In order to promote the general health of the community, without violating individual right to choose, I would consider implementing a variety of interventions to effectively reduce the consumption of processed meat. For example, educational initiatives, informative packaging, increasing taxes on the product, and liaising with companies to try and make the product healthier. **(solutions, if/then)** In summary, after gathering information to quantify the risk associated with consumption of processed meats as well as the actual risk posed to members of my community, I could move forward with a plan that protects individual health while respecting individual autonomy. **(summary)**

DISCUSSION: Though this question is discussing the implementation of a policy, it is a scenario question because it is asking you to act as a public health official and go through the steps you would take when deciding whether or not to implement the policy in your community. The "BAD" answer is brief, judgmental, and extreme. It does not include the steps that the individual would take when implementing such a policy. The "GOOD" answer approaches the question as a scenario question. The applicant starts off by identifying their main priorities and then goes about gathering information as they would if they were a public health official considering a new healthy policy. From there, they discuss the various solutions that they would implement to benefit their community, before concluding the prompt with a brief summary. This answer is clearly organized, and addresses the question posed in the prompt.

CASPer Scenario 8:

You are the manager in an office. Your team shares a common kitchen with a fridge. Some of your team members bring lunches with them to work and store them in the common fridge. Over the last couple of weeks various members of your team have noticed parts of their lunches are missing. More recently, entire lunches have been disappearing without a trace. Several upset team members have brought this issue to your attention.

1. What would do as the manager? (*ethical dilemma*)

2. Two of your team members, who sit near the lunchroom, have noticed the cleaning staff going in and out of the lunch room at odd hours, they want you to confront them. What would you say to your team members? (*conflict resolution, ethical dilemma*)

3. What would you say to the cleaning staff? (*conflict resolution, ethical dilemma*)

1. What would do as the manager?

BAD: This seems like a very minor issue. I would request that my team gets back to work and ignore any further requests to handle the issue. (**unempathetic**) I would encourage my team to focus on their work, which is the more important issue in this scenario. If further requests to handle the issue were made, then I would delegate the task to one of my employees so that I could focus on more important issues. (**unwilling to help others, or thinks they are above the hypothetical situation, red flag**)

GOOD: As the manager in this situation, my main priority would be the well-being of my team members, who are understandably distressed to find their lunches missing, as well as the well-being of the individual who is stealing lunches. **(identifying the most pressing issue)** I would start of by interviewing my team members, privately, in a non-confrontational manner to gather more information. It is possible that this is happening because someone on my team is going through difficult times financially or perhaps the cleaning staff are discarding the food thinking it has gone bad. I would also ask whether anyone had noticed suspicious behavior, but be careful about jumping to conclusions. **(information gathering)** If from my questioning, I discover that someone on my team is taking the lunches due to financial difficulties, I would point them to charities supplying free food to those in need or offer to help them with managing their budget by referring them to an expert in my network of friends and request that they not take from their co-workers without permission, because it is dishonest as well as unprofessional behavior. I might even consider looking into subsidized lunch initiatives, or having a communal snack area, for the whole team, to prevent this kind of behavior from occurring in the future. I would ask that this individual come to me if they are experiencing difficulties in the future, and make sure they understand that if this type of behavior continues, that they are at risk of losing their job, as it has been having a detrimental impact on our team. If my individual discussions did not yield any information as to the culprit, then I would hold a team meeting in the lunch room, explaining the situation and the steps I would be taking to prevent it. These steps might include installing security cameras in the lunch room, having a clearly marked communal snack area and a defined punishment for anyone caught stealing from their co-workers. I would reinforce that we are a team, and as such should not be stealing from one another, and that if anyone is having financial troubles, and is unable to afford food, then they are always welcome to come and talk to me about it. If, after these interventions, the theft continued, then I would have to unfortunately let the person responsible go, for their detrimental effect on the team dynamic. If however, it is resolved then no further action will be required on my part. **(solutions, if/then)** Thus, by gathering information about the situation from my team, I would be able to stop the theft, and protect the well-being of everyone involved while hopefully helping the perpetrator find other solutions. **(summary)**

DISCUSSION: In this scenario, you are a manager and you have been asked to handle an issue involving your team's lunches. In the "BAD" answer, the individual seems unwilling to deal with the issue. This is a huge red flag, and makes the candidate come across as entitled and unwilling to help others. This is not an acceptable answer. The "GOOD" answer follows the scenario question format. The applicant first gathers information from their employees, and then puts forward a variety of solutions that would both solve the problem and prevent the same problem from happening in the future. The answer shows depth of thought, empathy and good common sense decision making capabilities.

2. Two of your team members, who sit near the lunchroom, have noticed the cleaning staff going in and out of the lunch room at odd hours, they want you to confront them. What would you say to your team members?

BAD: I would tell my team that I will approach the cleaning staff and ask them if they have been stealing from the lunch room. It is unacceptable to have cleaning staff who steal from employees, and as such I would make sure that any individuals involved are immediately let go. This would stop the current thief and make future potential thieves think twice before stealing anything. Hopefully this would resolve the issue and reassure my team. **(extreme, judgemental, lacks depth of thought)**

GOOD: In this situation, I would want to address the concerns of my team members without alienating the cleaning staff by making them feel inappropriately persecuted. The primary objective is the well-being of my team including the cleaning staff. **(identifying the most pressing issue)** I would first talk to each of my team members privately to determine what exactly they saw, and why they were concerned about it. **(information gathering)** I would thank them for any information and reinforce that I am handling the situation and that I would appreciate their discretion in this matter. If my staff had only seen the cleaning staff coming in and out of the lunch room, carrying cleaning equipment and had not directly witnessed the cleaning staff stealing anything, then I would reassure my staff that it was likely part of the cleaning staff's regular duties. I would also reassure them that I will be speaking with the manager of the cleaning staff, to make him/her aware of the situation without accusing anyone and that in the meantime, I will continue to take action to try to find the true culprit. If, on the other hand, my staff had directly witnessed a member of the cleaning staff stealing food from our lunch room, then I would tell them that I will have a private conversation with that member of the staff and/or their manager, if a specific individual was not clearly identified. (**solutions, if/then**) By taking a non-judgemental approach and talking to all involved parties, I would hopefully be able to get to the bottom of this situation and prevent it from continuing to disrupt our work environment. (**summary**)

DISCUSSION: This prompt suggests that the cleaning staff may be responsible for the missing lunches. However, it is important to remember that you do not actually have evidence that the cleaning staff were stealing anything from the lunchroom. The "BAD" answer assumes that the employees are 100% correct in what they saw. It further assumes that the employees had witness the actual act of theft which is incorrect. The applicant does not consider that the cleaning staff may simply have been cleaning the lunch room, and immediately proceeds to dismiss them. It's important to conduct due diligence in this case and investigate the claims prior to jumping to conclusions. The "GOOD" answer follows the scenario question format and investigates the claims prior to providing a variety of solutions based on the various possibilities. The solutions offered in this answer are also less punitive, which makes the applicant appear non-judgemental and empathetic.

3. What would you say to the cleaning staff?

BAD: I would first schedule a meeting with the manager of the cleaning staff to discuss my concerns. I would disclose what had happened and report the individuals who were involved. Further, I would request that these individuals be fired as they are stealing from my employees. The act of stealing is unacceptable in the work place and is highly detrimental to the overall work environment. If the manager didn't agree with my assessment of the situation, then I would have to go above him, by either calling the police or talking to my own boss. I feel that this would be the right course of action, because my employees have a right to feel safe in the workplace. **(judgemental, unempathetic, did not gather information, extreme stance)**

GOOD: I would want to approach the cleaning staff in this situation, to get their side of the story by having a private conversion with each staff member. It is possible that my staff saw them performing their regular duties, and they are not involved in any way. **(non-judgemental)** My priority is to find the underlying cause of the situation without alienating anyone in the office or contributing to a negative work environment to ensure my team's well-being. **(identifying the most pressing issue)** Thus, I would first ask for a meeting with the manager of the cleaning staff to make him/her aware of the issue and see if he/she had any insight into the problem. **(information gathering)** I would also want to discuss any changes I would be making to the work environment to prevent further incidents that might impact cleaning. If my employees hadn't directly witnessed anyone stealing and the manager doesn't think his team was involved, then I will likely just ask them to make the cleaning staff aware of the problem and the ongoing changes and keep an eye out for any odd behavior. If, on the other hand, my staff or the manager have identified an individual who may be implicated in the situation, then I might also elect to talk to this member of the staff, either privately or with their manager present, to learn their side of the story. If it turns out that this person mistakenly thought the fridge was communal or had moved items accidentally, then I would ask them to avoid touching food while cleaning and monitor the situation by installing securing cameras, for example. If the person admits to stealing food due to financial hardship or other difficulties, I might point them to communal food resources within the company or community and give them one more chance, providing they understand the negative impact their actions had on my team and are remorseful. If the individual has been stealing food maliciously for whatever reason, then I would talk to the manager about having this individual dismissed, as they are purposefully creating a negative work environment. **(solutions, if/then)** In summary, a delicate approach is warranted in this situation to avoid alienating the cleaning staff through false accusations. By working with them and their manager to find out what is really happening, we could hopefully come to a resolution and prevent this issue from continuing to happen. **(summary)**

DISCUSSION: This question is now asking you to consider how you would approach the cleaning staff. Though it is valuable to talk to them to gain further insight into the situation, it must still be recognized that you do not have definitive proof that the cleaning staff are responsible. The "BAD" answer again assumes that the cleaning staff are responsible and suggests that anyone implicated should be fired, because they are a hazard to employee well-being and safety. Though employee well-being and safety are important in this scenario, the well-being of all employees, including the cleaning staff, should be considered. The "GOOD" answer addresses the prompt by gathering information from the manager of the cleaning staff as well as the staff themselves. By not jumping to conclusions, the applicant is able to work with the cleaning staff to resolve the problem. The various solutions presented demonstrate that the candidate has considered the various causes to the problem in this scenario and taken an empathetic approach to finding a solution that will result in the least amount of harm to all involved.

CASPer Scenario 9:

You are a professor at a university. After class one day, you are approached by a student you know who is asking you to write them a "strong" letter of recommendation for a professional program. The student has good grades in your course and asks you insightful questions during class. You have had several thoughtful discussions with him during your office hours, and quite enjoy talking to him. However, after spotting the student leaving your office one day last week, one of your colleagues approached you. She disclosed that the student had been caught plagiarizing assignments and cheating on exams in one of her courses last year. She claims that when she confronted him, he "threw a tantrum", stormed out of her office.

1. What would you say to the student? (*ethical dilemma*)

2. If you did write the letter, would you mention what your colleague had said about the student, why or why not? (*ethical dilemma*)

3. When selecting individuals for professional school, what do you think is more important: academic performance and standardized test scores or their ability to demonstrate professional-type behaviours across a variety of settings? (*policy*)

1. What would you say to the student?

BAD: My main concern in this situation is not recommending an inappropriate candidate for professional school, which could have a negative impact on society. (**judgemental without gathering more information, ignoring the well-being of the student**) Given what my colleague has told me, I am concerned about this student holding a position of power or one where he is interacting with the public. (**jumping to conclusions**) I know that if I refuse to write the letter, he will likely approach someone else for a letter. I am concerned that if that person is not aware of the situation, they may end up writing him a good letter. As such, I would agree to write him a letter, but make sure to include both my experiences with him and what I had heard about him from my colleague, because I want to make sure that the schools are aware of the type of applicant that they are getting. **(dishonest, red flag)**

GOOD: This would be a difficult situation to be in as a referee. I have a good relationship with this student, and not writing a letter of recommendation for him would definitely negatively impact his well-being and his future career. On the other hand, I am concerned about this report from my colleague, and would not want to recommend an unsuitable candidate for a professional school, as this could potentially negatively impact society, and possibly even my reputation. **(values)** Before agreeing to write the student a letter, I would have to explain what I had heard about the situation to him and ask him for his perspective. I would also seek to clarify the incident further with my colleague. **(information gathering)** It is possible that I misunderstood or misheard my colleague, in which case I would have no problem writing the letter. It is also possible that the student did react this way but was also facing multiple stressors in his personal life that, while not excusing the bad behavior, may indicate it was an acute stress reaction rather than a pervasive worrisome character trait. **(empathy)** In this case, I would consider writing the letter, assuming the student demonstrated adequate reflective abilities indicating that he had worked on his coping skills and learned from the unfortunate incident. If the student denied the incident or had another angry outburst when I brought it up, and talking to my colleague had confirmed my suspicions, then I would have to tell him that I was honestly concerned about the behavior pattern and would thus be unable to write him a "strong" reference letter. **(solutions, if/then)** By talking to the student and taking his perspective into account, as well as clarifying the issue with my colleague, I would be able to resolve the situation in a way that is fair to the student, while protecting society from the potentially harmful effects of unsuitable candidates gaining entry into professional schools. **(summary)**

DISCUSSION: The key components of solving the problem presented in this stem are determining what really happened in your colleague's office, determining why it happened, and then having an honest discussion with the student about whether you will write him a reference letter. This question is looking at what you would say to the student. The "BAD" answer acts on the assumption that everything you ascertained from a brief hallway conversation with your colleague is correct. Given the negative impact of writing a bad letter, the possibility that your initial interpretation of the story was incorrect must at least be investigated. Deliberately lying to the student about the quality of the letter is also unethical. On the other hand, the "GOOD" answer is first able to determine the most pressing issues which include a combination of the well-being of your students, the general public and even the professor's own reputation. Further the applicant takes the time to gather more information before making a decision. Finally, the applicant verbalizes possible solutions based on our "if/then" strategy making sure the final decision shows empathy, sound judgement and least amount of harm to those involved.

2. If you did write the letter, would you mention what your colleague had said about the student, why or why not?

BAD: My main concern in this scenario is not recommending an inappropriate candidate for professional school. (**values, ignoring well-being of the student, unempathetic**) In this case, I would mention what my colleague had said, because I am concerned about this student's violent behavior. (**jumping to conclusions**) This type of behavior would be completely inappropriate in a professional and, as such, I feel that it is something important for schools to know prior to accepting him. Further, I would worry that if I told him that the letter would not be "strong", he may simply go an ask someone else for a reference letter. Hence, to ensure that an inappropriate candidate is not admitted, and thus to protect society, I would agree to write the "strong" letter and include a note of the outburst that my colleague had witnessed in the letter.

GOOD: The question indicates that the student was asking for a "strong" reference letter. If I did write a letter including the incident that my colleague disclosed, it would negatively reflect on the student, and could have a huge negative impact by preventing him from entering professional school and limiting his future career options. **(identifying most pressing issue)** Further, reference letters are supposed to be based on direct interactions and observations of the student, so it would likely be unfair to include any "hearsay" from a colleague, especially given that my personal interactions with this student have always been pleasant. At the same time, I would not want to recommend an inappropriate and potentially unprofessional candidate who may abuse the trust and power granted to him by society. **(values, identifying pressing issues)** Thus, I would first have to gather more information by having a private conversion with the student, my colleague and anyone else who may be familiar with the incident. **(information gathering)** If I had determined what my colleague had said to be true beyond a reasonable doubt (i.e.: had objective evidence of the incident) and the student had demonstrated a similar pattern of volatility during our interactions or was unable to offer me a reasonable explanation for the outburst, or had a history of repeated outbursts, I would be concerned about his ability to act as a professional. If this was the case, I would tell him honestly that I didn't think he was a suitable candidate, based on his behavior, and that I would thus be unable to write him a "strong" reference letter. If, even after this frank discussion, he still requested a reference letter from me, I would agree, but I would make sure he understood that it would be honest and include all of my observations, both positive and negative, about his behavior. On the other hand, if I find that the incident was isolated, due to some personal issues at the time, or perhaps my colleague was in the wrong, then I would gladly write a positive reference letter for the student. **(solutions, if/then)** By remaining objective about the situation, gathering more facts and only including an honest account of my direct observations about the student's behavior, I would be able to write him a fair letter while doing my due diligence to society. **(summary)**

DISCUSSION: There are several factors at play in this scenario. You heard a rumor from your colleague about this individual but are not completely sure of its validity. Including false information in his reference letter could destroy the student's chances of being accepted into professional school and have a significant detrimental effect on his overall well-being and future career options. On the other hand, you don't want to recommend an inappropriate, and allegedly unethical, individual to a professional school. You may be concerned about the potential impact this might have on society. Further, he has asked you for a strong reference letter, and it would be unethical for you to lie to him about the quality of the letter. The "BAD" answer does just this, and agrees to write the student a letter, without disclosing to him that it will not be the "strong" letter he is expecting. Lying to the student is unethical and will be a red flag to the CASPer raters. In addition, referees are generally asked to include information from their own observations of the student. This answer does not consider the well-being of the candidate or the need for at least confirming that the information is true before including it. The "GOOD" answer gives the well-being of the candidate fair consideration and does not assume that the rumors they heard from their colleague are true. Instead, this applicant gathers information from various sources in an effort to learn more about the situation and then is honest with the student about the quality of the letter.

3. When selecting individuals for professional school, what do you think is more important: academic performance and standardized test scores or their ability to demonstrate professional-type behaviors across a variety of settings?

BAD: When selecting candidates for professional school, I believe that academics are more important than the candidates' ability to demonstrate professional behavior. **(extreme stance)** First of all, academic scores, such as GPAs or standardized test scores, are more objective. Basing candidate selection from objective criteria is fair, and further, it is the only way to ensure that the very best candidates are selected. In addition, professional school is often difficult, and having minimum academic requirements ensures that the selected students are up to the task. **(narrow thought process, neglects the disadvantages of using academic scores, doesn't address professional skills)**

GOOD: I believe that both the applicants' academic performance, and their ability to act professionally across a variety of settings should be considered. **(addressing the prompt, non-judgemental)** Academic performance and standardized test scores, while not a good indicator of character, are a quick and easy way for professional schools to determine whether a candidate can successfully handle the academic rigors of their program and the cognitive load of the profession. Research has indicated that it is significantly easier to rehabilitate a student who has had an academic lapse than it is to rehabilitate a student who has lapsed professionally, and that students with professional lapses are significantly less likely to complete the program successfully than their peers. Furthermore, test scores have been correlated with bias against low income individuals while not being correlated with future on-the-job behavior. **(demonstrates specific knowledge of topic, addresses pros and cons)** One could, of course, argue that students who are already in a professional school have been screened based on their academic performance and standardized test scores, and are thus likely highly intelligent. As such an academic lapse is more likely caused by a transient external factor (such as an illness) than a lack of ability to carry the course load, making them significantly easier to remediate. Professional behaviors, on the other hand, are difficult to screen. Further, it is difficult to extrapolate how a student will react to the stresses placed on them by a professional school from the tools available to admissions committees today, namely essays and brief interviews. Applicants usually know that they are being tested on professionalism and again those coming from high income families have been shown to do better on professionalism tests. Unprofessional behaviors may be a product of a consistently stressful environments, unfamiliarity with the cultural norms of the western society or of the candidates themselves. **(further pros and cons)** Thus, though academics and professional behaviors both are important, in my opinion, if professional schools wish to address the problem of unprofessionalism and prevent professional lapses, they should pay more attention to professional behaviors across a variety of settings when selecting candidates and develop better tools for screening for professionalism, without causing implicit bias against applicants from lower income families. This will help select applicants who are better suited for their future professions, experience job satisfaction, and display reduced levels of burnout and professional misconduct. **(alternative solutions)**

DISCUSSION: This question is a policy type question, examining the nuances of admission to professional schools. For this question, one may choose to either showcase their knowledge of the issue, by discussing current events or research, or, to use a personal narrative to explore the issue. This helps to add weight and substance to the answer, while making it more memorable. The "BAD" answer fails to cite any evidence, through personal experience or knowledge of the issue, and only presents only a one-sided discussion of the issue. It lacks maturity of thought and broad perspective. The "GOOD" answer discusses both sides of the issue and uses knowledge of current events to back up their reasoning. They acknowledge that both are important but suggest which one schools should focus on more and offers a logical solution based on their previous discussion of the issue. Note how the applicant addressed this policy type question using our framework, without ever explicitly using "pros and cons" or similar phrases? This is what we want you to do eventually. Initially, it's O.K. to use our frameworks and use them verbatim but once you get the process and see the pattern, start using your own works while adhering to our strategies.

CASPer Scenario 10:

You work as a server at a busy restaurant. On this particular day, you are at least 30 minutes behind in the kitchen, meaning that customers are becoming disgruntled. At your last staff meeting, the manager specifically requested that you all do your best to avoid getting this far behind, as it forces them to turn customers away, thus negatively impacting the restaurant's revenue. As you are picking up a finished plate, you notice that it is covered in cheese, when the customer specifically requested "No Dairy". You point this out to the cook, who curses and then quickly picks off the cheese and re-fluffs the dish to hide any remaining pieces.

1. What would you say to the cook, who is technically your senior? (*ethical dilemma*)

2. What would you say to the customer? (*ethical dilemma*)

3. How have you managed conflict with a superior in the past? (*personal question, conflict resolution*)

1. What would you say to the cook, who is technically your senior?

BAD: In this scenario, I would be most concerned with the health and well-being of the customer. As such, I would notify the cook that picking the cheese off the plate was not good enough in this situation. If the person has a dairy allergy, small pieces of cheese could cause an anaphylactic reaction or worse. Plus, if the cook put on cheese, he may have forgotten to leave out dairy in the other components of the meal. Thus, to protect the safety of the customer, I would tell the cook to re-make the meal as quickly as possible. (**judgemental, lack of information gathering**)

GOOD: I would start off by acknowledging the fact that we are a busy service and behind tonight. I know from personal experience working in the restaurant industry, how much extra time it can take to prepare an allergen free meal properly, and how busy the kitchen can get. (**empathy**) However, in this situation, I would prioritize the safety of the customer over the efficiency of the kitchen. (**identifying the most pressing issue**) Though getting behind could negatively impact the company's bottom line in the short term, harming a customer could have long lasting negative repercussions both for us and the individual. (**considering multiple implications, weighing values**) Before making a decision, I would first have a quick conversation with the customer to find out if they have any food allergies or any other reasons that would prevent them from enjoying their meal if their plate had accidentally touched dairy. If they say, that it's not a problem, then I would serve their food and no further action is necessary. On the other hand, if the customer indicates that they have a severe allergy or for whatever reason they would not be able to consume their meal if the plate has contacted dairy, then I would apologize to them about the inadvertent accident and the delay and that we would be preparing their meal right away again. Furthermore, I would speak to the cook to let him know that we must prepare the dish again and offer to help if they are overwhelmed in the kitchen by talking to our manager and asking for other staff to join us during this shift. **(solutions, if/then)** In this way, I can make sure that the customer is safe while at the same time we are able to meet our revenue expectations without compromising the quality of our services.

DISCUSSION: The key to this question is recognizing the potential for harm to the customer and balancing that with the financial needs of the company. The stem does not specify whether the customer is avoiding dairy due to allergy, intolerance, or personal preference, so a good first step would be talking to the customer and determining their preference. As a restaurant or server, it would be unacceptable to knowingly give someone with a dairy allergy food containing dairy, so, if this information could not be gathered, it would be advisable to always err on the side of caution and just remake the dish. The "BAD" answer recognizes the risk to the well-being of the customer but does not do a good job of addressing the prompt, in terms of outlining what they would do to gather more information before deciding. It also lacks maturity of thought and shows an inability to recognize the broader implications and alternatives. The "GOOD" answer shows an applicant who is empathetic with the cook and does her best to make sure that no harm comes to the customer while minimizing delay in the kitchen by actually asking the customer why they requested no dairy and what they would prefer. They also address other ways in which they would help the cook catch up, indicating that they are both empathetic and a team player through their problem solving.

2. What would you say to the customer?

BAD: I would approach the customer's table to tell them that their meal would be taking longer than expected as the cook had made an error. **(judgemental, lack of information gathering)** If they are upset about the situation, I could offer a food or drink discount after talking to the manager and explaining to him what the cook had done. **(lack of empathy, narrow minded)** I might also inform him about the cook's lack of attention to detail **(judgemental)** and concern for the well-being of the customer.

GOOD: I would approach the customer, explain what had happened, apologize, and inform them how long the cook had said it would take to get a new dish. I would then ask them if they had a severe allergy, and if not, would they rather we remake the dish or just serve it as is, even though it is contaminated with a small amount of cheese. **(information gathering)** If they had an allergy or were really opposed to eating dairy for any reason, but were understanding about the extra time, then I would report back to the cook, telling him we would have to remake the dish, and helping him to do so as needed. If they didn't have an allergy and didn't mind a bit of contamination, then I would simply bring them the dish. If they didn't want to wait for a new dish, I might offer them another, faster, dairy free dish. If they weren't interested in that, I would apologize again, ask if there was anything else I could bring and make sure to remove the item from their bill. **(solutions, if then)** By being honest with the customer in this situation, I would be able to keep him safe, while doing my best to keep the kitchen on time. **(summary)**

DISCUSSION: This question is now asking how you would deal with the customer. The important steps here would include communicating what had happened, apologizing, and finding a solution to the problem based on the customer's needs. In the "BAD" question, there is no discussion with the customer about how they would like the situation handled. Further, after assuming about what the customer will want, the applicant goes on to blame the cook for what happened. The stem never actually said who was to blame for the error, it only said that the customer had requested "No Dairy", so the situation may not have been the cook's fault. Taking it a step further and reporting the incident to management may also be a presumptive escalation. If one did want to discuss reporting the cook to the manager, they should likely also outline that they were certain the cook was responsible for the error, had made similar errors repeatedly in the past, and consistently showed a lack of remorse. If this was the case, it would be reasonable to report this person, as they are clearly at risk of causing serious harm to a customer, which is unacceptable. The "GOOD" answer does not jump to conclusions about who is at fault in the situation. Instead of laying blame, this applicant apologizes to the customer, determines what their preference is, and provides solutions based on that preference. The applicant shows a broader consideration of the situation, that takes all competing issues into account.

3. How have you managed conflict with a superior in the past?

BAD: I recently had a conflict with a superior over vacation time. My sister, who I hadn't seen in over a year, was coming to visit from Australia, and I requested 2 days off to spend time visiting with her. I didn't think that it would be a big issue, because one of my coworkers had recently gotten a month off to travel to Guatemala. To my surprise, my boss refused to give me any time off to visit with my sister. I was very disappointed and went to his office to discuss the issue. He acknowledged that it did seem unfair, given that my co-worker had recently gotten so much time off, but he felt that giving my co-worker that much time off had been a poor managerial choice, as my co-worker had abused the privilege and not completed his work obligations while away. Further, he informed me that the company would be changing their time off policy, which was disappointing because it had been a big benefit of working for them. **(red flag, the applicant admits to working a job mostly due to vacation benefits)** I managed to reach a compromise with him, and secured one day off, though he informed me that I would still be expected to come in the other day. I did come in the second day, but felt very resentful, and purposefully did little work during my shift to make a point. (**immature response**) Me not doing my work that day really made no difference. (**poor sentence structure, remember, raters are humans and they do care even if they are told not to care about grammar and spelling**) The situation taught me that sometimes managers don't make the best decisions. (**judgemental**) In the future, I will try to work with people who don't take out their issues with other employees on me and who acknowledge the hard work that I put in for their company. (**not a lot of individual learning**)

GOOD: I recently had a conflict with a superior over vacation time. (**recap**) My sister, who I hadn't seen in over a year, was coming to visit from Australia, and I requested 2 days off to spend time visiting with her. I didn't think that it would be a big issue, because one of my coworkers had recently gotten a month off to travel to Guatemala. To my surprise, my boss refused to give me any time off to spend with my sister. I was very disappointed and went to his office to discuss the issue with him privately. He acknowledged that it did seem unfair, given that my co-worker had recently gotten so much time off, but he felt that giving my co-worker that much time off had been a poor managerial choice, as my co-worker had abused the privilege and not completed his work obligations while away. Further, he informed me that the company would be changing their time off policy, which was not a problem because I actually enjoy working there and I wasn't there just for vacation time. By explaining how important it was to me to be able to see my sister, I managed to reach a compromise with him by assuring that I would get all of my work done early, before I took the time off. This meant I had to work a bit harder for the two weeks before my sister visited, but it was worth it, as I was able to reach my work obligations and visit with my sister. My ability to get my work done on time also helped to rebuild trust with my manager, who decided to re-instate my flexible vacation policy based on my strong work ethic. (**positive outcome**) Though it wasn't a great experience for me at the time, because I didn't get to spend as much time with my sister as I would have liked, the situation taught me that hard work and dedication do pay off eventually. In addition, because I was able to prove to my manager that I could be trusted to work remotely, I was later allowed to visit my sister in Australia for 3 weeks during our slow season. (**what I learned, positive outcome**) In the future, I hope to continue to use my dedication and strong work ethic to build trust with those who I work with and to use communication to reach mutually acceptable solutions in similarly challenging situations. (**future application**)

DISCUSSION: This is a personal question examining how the candidate deals with conflict. In the "BAD" answer, the applicant shows an immature response to a disappointment, which could be a red flag. Further, it reveals that the applicant had been in a job primarily because of its vacation policy rather than the desire to be part of the team and enjoy the job itself. The "GOOD" answer shows a different response to the same situation. In this example, the candidate responded to a seemingly unfair managerial decision by working to earn back the manager's trust. Their ability to balance both work and their time off shows good time management skills, and the positive outcome demonstrates that they were able to demonstrate to the manager that they are worthy of their trust. Further, the applicant shows that they are not concerned about the changes to the vacation policy because they love their job, rather they are more concerned about not being able to spend time with their sister. By showing a positive outcome, framing the experience in a positive way, and choosing an experience that offered an opportunity for growth, this applicant was able to showcase their more mature response to the situation. The applicant understands that even seemingly challenging situations can be resolved with communication, flexibility, and that trust.

CASPer Scenario 11:

> "*Success is walking from failure to failure with no loss of enthusiasm.*"
>
> -- Winston Churchill

1. What is your interpretation of Winston Churchill's quote? (*personal*)

2. Would you change anything about the quote, if you could? (*personal*)

3. Describe a time in your life when you failed. (*personal*)

1. What is your interpretation of Winston Churchill's quote?

BAD: To me, the quote means that success is all about not giving up in the face of failure. Basically, if you don't succeed, the most important thing is to continue to try. **(brief, lacks personal account)**

GOOD: To me, Winston Churchill's quote is meant to remind us that perfection is not a pre-requisite for being successful in life, that behind most successful individuals lies a long string of failures, and that what eventually made them successful was that they kept trying. **(summary and interpretation of the quote)** This lesson is exemplified almost any time you learn a new skill or work towards a goal. Recently this lesson was re-enforced for me through my gradual come back from a long-standing running injury. Through a combination of life stress and lack of strength training, I managed to give myself bilateral glute tendonitis as well as a tendonitis in my peroneal tendon. **(personal example, problem)** Both of these injuries are known for their long recovery times, and when I first visited my physiotherapist, close to tears with frustration, she implored me to be patient and not give up. Working with her, I learned a variety of exercises, and did them faithfully as prescribed, despite limited improvement. I did mind numbing pool and elliptical work to maintain my fitness, but as time wore on, my motivation waned. Still my exercises didn't work, the expensive massages and acupuncture treatments didn't work. Even though I was able to walk pain free, every time I tried to run, the pain came back. My friends and family told me to give it a rest. Frustrated, I decided to switch my focus, instead of trying to run and repeatedly re-injuring myself I would just try to heal. I would keep doing the things recommended by my physiotherapist, because I was seeing mild improvement. However, it was evident we were missing something, and I made it my mission to find out what. So, I threw myself into learning everything I could about both conditions, testing some differentials and methodically trying every trick in the book until I got to the root of the problem. Though a lot of things didn't work, slowly, I stumbled upon techniques that did and added them to my repertoire. **(solution)** Soon, the pain went away. Then, I began to run, slowly at first, the sharp pain now a niggle. Eventually, I worked my way back up to half my normal mileage, then ¾. In less than two months, I will return to racing. **(positive outcome)** I will be slower than I was before the injuries, but thanks to all the rehab, much stronger. The experience taught me the value of maintaining a positive attitude in the face of repeated setbacks. **(what was learned)** In the future, when I come head to head with repeated failures and feel like giving up, I will remember this experience and how maintaining a positive outlook and trying new things allowed me to achieve my goal and come back stronger then I was before. **(apply to future)**

DISCUSSION: This is a personal question asking you to interpret the meaning of the quote provided. The "BAD" answer provides a very brief interpretation of the meaning of the quote. Though the interpretation is not wrong, this applicant has missed an opportunity to make their answer more memorable by telling a personal story detailing a time they refused to give up. Using a personal narrative also will allow you to showcase some of your strengths and experiences. The "GOOD" answer does just this, by utilizing a memorable personal narrative about overcoming injury. The narrative is applicable to the quote and tells a story of triumph despite repeated failures. The applicant summarizes their response by detailing what they learned and how they will apply that lesson in the future.

2. Would you change anything about the quote, if you could?

BAD: One of my favorite quotes is the quote often attributed to Albert Einstein "Insanity is doing the same thing over and over and expecting different results". If I were to amend Winston Churchill's quote, it would be to add something about the importance of using each failed attempt as a learning experience.

(brief, lacks personal account, doesn't explain why they would amend it in this way)

GOOD: One of my favorite quotes is the quote often attributed to Albert Einstein "Insanity is doing the same thing over and over and expecting different results". If I were to amend Winston Churchill's quote, it would be to add something about the importance of using each failed attempt as a learning experience. **(intro addresses the question)** For example, I was not successful the first time I tried to do an intravenous injection on a dummy. The doctor teaching me gave me feedback on where I went wrong on each attempt, which I then applied to the subsequent attempt. By modifying my technique according to what I learned with each attempt, I was eventually able to get the IV on my first try every time. This experience of gradually incorporating feedback from multiple attempts allowed me to develop the skill required and engage in troubleshooting for myself when errors did occur. Each failure taught me something new about the procedure, which I then applied to subsequent attempts. **(personal example)** Learning something from each failure helped to develop my expertise and made me feel confident that I could do this skill in a variety of settings in the future. **(why it's important)** Thus, I would modify the quote to include the importance of not only not giving up in the face of failure, but also seeking to learn from it by getting expert feedback on my performance. **(summary)**

(Important note here: this of course also applies to you as you learn how to think and behave professionally, both in life and your CASPer test. The best and only way to learn a new skill is not by practicing it mindlessly, rather by deliberate practice while seeking expert feedback, as discussed earlier.)

DISCUSSION: This question is asking the applicant if they would change the quote in any way. Both the "GOOD" and the "BAD" example opt to improve the quote by including the importance of learning from one's failures, however the "BAD" example doesn't explain why they think that this would be a valuable modification to make. The "GOOD" example uses a relevant personal narrative to illustrate their point, thus making their answer more personable and demonstrating why they think this would be an important addition.

3. Describe a time in your life where you "failed".

BAD: Something in life that I consistently fail at is being a perfectionist. For me, being a perfectionist means spending too much time on unimportant tasks, because I feel that everything has to be done "right". Often, I procrastinate on tasks because I am overwhelmed by the effort it will take to do them correctly. **(generic response, non-specific examples)** In this way, my perfectionism holds me back. **(lacks solutions, sounds cliché)**

GOOD: Recently, I failed to receive an interview for an internship that I was really excited about. **(addressing question)** Rather than get discouraged, I decided to keep applying to other internships that, though seemed less desirable, would still help me to build my skill sets for a position as staff writer for a national health magazine. **(turning it into positive action)** I did succeed in securing one of those positions, and by working hard and constantly asking for feedback from my manager, I learned a lot from the position. The company liked my attitude and work so much that they eventually offered me a full-time position, which has given me even more opportunities to build my skill set and I learned even more than I would have with the original internship. **(positive outcome from action)** This experience taught me that although you may not always get exactly what you want, by maintaining a positive attitude, being enthusiastic, and continuing to seek enjoyable learning opportunities, you can discover even better opportunities that you may not have known existed. **(what was learned)** In the future, I will continue to look at disappointments, not as failures, but as opportunities to expand my horizons and approach problems from a novel perspective. **(future applications)**

DISCUSSION: This is a personal question asking the applicant to describe a time in their life when they failed. The "BAD" answer fails to discuss a specific instance of when the failure occurred. As a result, it is difficult for the reader to ascertain what was learned from the situation. In addition, being "a perfectionist" is a very common answer, meaning that this one will not stand out. The "GOOD" answer uses a specific example of a time the applicant failed. The applicant discusses what they did in response to the failure and frames it as a learning opportunity, by talking about the positive outcome and what they learned from the situation.

CASPer Scenario 12:

Social media has become an integral part of our society and has changed both how we view the world and how we interact with one another. Recently, however, we are seeing the dark side of social media. For example, a private corporation recently admitted to the use of private users' data by one of its clients to sway public opinion during a major election.

1. What are some other ways in which widespread social media use, and the resulting data collection, could negatively impact our society? (*policy, cons*)

2. How can widespread social media use and data collection benefit our society? (*policy, pros*)

3. How can we better protect members of the public from the misuse of their private data? (*policy, alternatives*)

1. What are some other ways in which widespread social media use, and the resulting data collection, could negatively impact our society?

BAD: Widespread social media use and the resulting data collection has a decidedly negative impact on our society. Doctored pictures of "Instagram models" create unrealistic body image expectations, causing body dissatisfaction, low self-esteem and eating disorders. Further, people tend to portray only "good times" on social media, creating a selection bias that causes individuals to feel that their lives pale in comparison to that of their peers. **(narrow thought process, only considers psychological issues related to sharing images)** In conclusion, widespread social media is likely responsible for the high rates of mental health issues that we see in youth today. **(unsupported, judgemental conclusion)**

GOOD: There are several ways in which widespread social media use could negatively impact our society. **(recap)** This could occur not only through inappropriate data collection, as mentioned in the question, but also through some of the documented negative health and mental health effects associated with extensive social media use. **(broader implications)** There are many ways in which inappropriate data collection could negatively impact individuals. For instance, inappropriately sharing activity or health data with health insurance companies could result in widespread denial of health insurance to applicants. Inappropriate collection of information by corporations and the government could result in widespread violation of individual right to privacy. Widespread social media has been shown to negatively impact our mental and physical health in a variety of ways. For instance, the doctored images that frequently appear in social media can contribute to the development of unrealistic expectations surrounding body shape and size. Further, people tend to portray only "good times" on social media, creating a selection bias that causes individuals to feel that their lives pale in comparison to that of their peers. Finally, too much time on social media can detract from the time that individuals spend exercising or socializing. This can have significant negative benefits on both their physical and mental health. **(negative impacts)** Thus, social media and data collection should be regulated to ensure that individual privacy is protected, and that the negative impacts to individual physical, mental and social well-being are minimized. **(summary)**

DISCUSSION: This question is asking about the negative impact of social media and widespread data collection in our society. This question focuses on the disadvantages only and therefore it is similar to when addressing the disadvantages in a policy type question. The "BAD" answer only considers the negative psychological impacts of social media use, and does not provide any consideration of the negative impacts that social media use may have on physical health or social well-being. Further, this answer did not address the negative impacts of data collection. In addition, the conclusion made did not follow from the facts presented in the body of the answer. This answer could have been improved by taking a broader approach and using facts to back up the conclusion. The "GOOD" answer provides a more thorough consideration of the negative impacts associated with both social media use and widespread data collection. Consideration is given to many aspects of an individual's well-being, including their physical, social, and emotional health. Overall, this answer shows a broad consideration of all the issues and makes several well-informed points. The answer is also well organized, with a mapping statement, list of points and concluding sentence.

2. How can widespread social media use and data collection benefit our society?

BAD: A lot of studies have shown the negative impacts of social media on the mental health of teens. Teens may feel a lot of pressure to behave or look a certain way knowing that it is likely they will be featured on social media. This can create a lot of social anxiety and other issues. Overall, social media does not have a lot of positive impacts on our society and our ancestors lives without social media just fine. **(lacks maturity of thought, judgemental, extreme, one-sided)**

GOOD: Widespread social media use and data collection has the potential to benefit our individuals and society in various ways. **(recap)** There are in fact several ways in which widespread social media use and data collection could benefit both individuals and society in terms of physical health, safety, and individual's ability to connect with one another socially. For instance, the widespread collection and study of health-related data could allow public health officials to learn more about the main contributors to mental and physical disease within our society. Data mined from videos shared on social media can also be valuable for solving crimes or locating people of interest, thus helping with law enforcement efforts. Collecting personal health data through devices can also help to expedite diagnosis or management of specific health conditions, for instance, in some individuals who have abnormal heart rhythms, continuous monitoring through wrist-based devices can help to give their doctors more information relevant for diagnosis and treatments. Social media can be used to promote freedom of speech when they are not censored. Finally, social media use can also have positive social benefits, by connecting individuals without geographical boundaries, making it easier to organize groups and keeping individuals informed on relevant social initiatives. **(positive points)** Thus, social media and widespread data collection can positively impact the lives of both individuals and society by facilitating data collection on individual and public health, promoting freedom of speech, increasing public safety, and facilitating social connections. **(summary/conclusion)**

DISCUSSION: This question is asking about the positive impacts of social media and widespread data collection in our society. This question focuses on the advantages only and therefore it is similar to when addressing the pros in a policy type question. The "BAD" answer doesn't address the positive aspects of social media use or data collection, and thus fails to answer the question. There is also no consideration of how widespread data collection could benefit individuals or society. The "GOOD" answer provides a more thorough consideration of the positive impacts associated with both social media use and widespread data collection. Thorough consideration is given to the benefits of widespread data collection and how it can improve individuals' health and safety. The answer is also well organized, with a mapping statement, list of points and concluding sentence.

3. How can we better protect members of the public from the misuse of their private data?

BAD: Members of the public should protect themselves from data misuse. Limiting the amount of information they disclose online, limiting the time spent online and avoiding interacting with strangers online are all good ways to maintain anonymity and avoid security breaches. Further, individuals should be careful when making online purchases or sharing credit card information online. By being wary of sharing and only disclosing information when necessary, individuals should be able to protect themselves more effectively. **(lacks maturity of thought, only explores individual culpability)**

GOOD: There are a variety of things we could do to help better protect the public from misuse of their private data. **(recap)** Educating the public about the risks and how to ascertain whether an online source can be trusted or not would be a good first step. More importantly, the corporations who collect the data themselves, such as social media sites, should have stringent regulations placed upon them in terms of the conditions under which they collect and share data. Consent should always be obtained from the individuals from whom data is being collected, and the purpose of data collection should be clear. Collected data should always be anonymized, so that individuals cannot be tracked, and their privacy is protected. Finally, the government should regulate which groups can have access to social media data, keeping in mind the benefit (or lack thereof) that these groups provide to society and the public at large. Ideally, these transactions should be monitored by a third-party regulatory body who has the public's best interests at heart to ensure transparency and adherence to guidelines set out by the government. **(alternative solutions)** By educating the public, increasing the regulations on corporations, and employing a third-party regulatory body, we could increase the safety of online activity while minimizing the risk for harm or data misuse. **(summary)**

DISCUSSION: This question is delving into the issues surrounding online security and the proper management of public data. It focuses on the other possible solutions and therefore it is like addressing the alternative solutions in a policy type question. To address this question, one must consider the various areas in which data breaches can occur as well as how risk can be mitigated. The "BAD" answer puts the onus on the individual to protect themselves. This strategy is unlikely to work, as individuals may not recognize the risks they are taking when sharing personal data online, and it can be very difficult to effect behavioral change at the individual level. Furthermore, individuals are not able to control how third parties use their personal information. No consideration to regulation at the corporate or government level is given, showing a very narrow perspective. The "GOOD" answer considers what individuals can do to protect themselves as well as how corporations and the government can act to address the problem. This shows a deeper understanding of the processes at work and a broader perspective.

Now that we have outlined our step-by-step strategies and have provided you with multiple examples of GOOD versus BAD responses, it is time to apply what you learned. The next chapter, which includes the equivalent of two CASPer practice tests, will allow you to apply the BeMo strategies. Before you start, re-read the previous chapter first. Here is what we want you to do. For the first set, do *not* time yourself, rather go over each scenario and practice by identifying the question types and applying the BeMo framework for acing any CASPer question outlined in *Chapter VI: 17 Proven Strategies to Prepare for and Ace Any CASPer Test* before formulating your response. Then get expert feedback from a mature professional (or sign up for a BeMo CASPer prep program) so you can learn from your mistakes. It is critical that you do not rely on feedback from your peers or students in the field because, students, even though accepted in your program of choice are not qualified to provide mentorships and often have not yet developed the insight to accurately assess your performance. For this reason, BeMo almost never hires students in training as admissions experts.

Once you are completely satisfied and confident that you got all the questions in the first practice test, it's time to write your second practice test. This time however, we want you to do it a bit differently by timing yourself and treating the test like an actual test by typing your responses on the same computer you will be using to write your actual test in the same exact location, and even at the same time as your scheduled test time, while wearing the same outfit you will be wearing during test date. Give yourself exactly 5 minutes to answer all three questions for each scenario. Write the test in one sitting and do not go back and modify any of your answers. Furthermore, give yourself a 15-minute break after you have completed scenario #6 to mimic the actual test. Once you have written the test, go back and look at your responses and our formula to find out what you think you did well and what you think you did poorly. Then, as always, seek expert feedback.

CHAPTER IX

Sample CASPer Practice Tests

CASPer Practice Test I

CASPer Scenario 1:

You are a university student. A close friend is starting a new student organization that seeks to highlight and celebrate achievements of citizens of European-descent. Your friend hopes to teach colleagues about history and celebrate the country's heritage. Your classmate Lucia finds out about this and is visibly uncomfortable. She perceives this as a direct attack on all non-Caucasian students whose families may be recent immigrants to the country.

1. How will you approach this situation?

2. What issues are important to keep in mind?

3. Describe a time when you helped resolve a conflict between two friends or acquaintances.

What type(s) of CASPer scenario is this?

What's the most pressing issue?

What are the missing facts?

Who is directly and indirectly involved?

What are some possible solutions using if/then strategy?

CASPer Scenario 2:

Your friend Allie is in her last year of dental school. She occasionally posts "before and after" pictures of her patients' teeth on social media. She never includes names, and there is no way to identify the patient in question from the picture. Her last caption read: "Took care of this foul mouth today: three cavities and an abscess. Come on people, please have better mouth hygiene!"

1. What is going through your mind right now?

2. How would you act in this situation?

3. Describe a time when something inappropriate was posted on social media and how you responded.

<u>What type(s) of CASPer scenario is this?</u>

<u>What's the most pressing issue?</u>

<u>What are the missing facts?</u>

Who is directly and indirectly involved?

What are some possible solutions using if/then strategy?

CASPer Scenario 3:

You have just started doing research at a prestigious neuroscience lab. This lab studies the effect of Lysergic Acid Diethylamide (LSD) micro-dosing on mice brains. This psychedelic drug may have ground-breaking applications for patients suffering from depression. Over time, you become more involved in the research and your lab Principal Investigator (PI) trusts you to obtain the drug for the lab. At this moment, you are made aware that all drugs are obtained illegally from a well-known criminal in your community.

1. What would you do in this situation?

2. What if your PI explains that there is no other way to obtain the drug for the experiments, and that this research could eventually save millions of lives?

3. In your opinion, do ends ever justify the means?

What type(s) of CASPer scenario is this?

What's the most pressing issue?

What are the missing facts?

Who is directly and indirectly involved?

What are some possible solutions using if/then strategy?

CASPer Scenario 4:

You are a university student. One evening, you find yourself "googling" your political science professor, who you strongly admire. You come across her profile on a review website. You click through the reviews your professor wrote for restaurants and other businesses along the years and are shocked to read racist and homophobic remarks in some of her reviews. This is particularly surprising because she appears kind and fair in class.

1. What would you do?

2. What if she begs you not to discuss or show these reviews with the university, and vows to erase them immediately?

3. Discuss a time when someone you admired disappointed you.

<u>What type(s) of CASPer scenario is this?</u>

<u>What's the most pressing issue?</u>

<u>What are the missing facts?</u>

<u>Who is directly and indirectly involved?</u>

<u>What are some possible solutions using if/then strategy?</u>

CASPer Scenario 5:

You are taking a university history class with your best friend, Janine. Throughout the semester, you notice the Teaching Assistant (T.A.), a graduate student who grades all assignments and exams, gets progressively friendlier with Janine. You even think they may be flirting. One afternoon, you find them behind the university building embracing and kissing. You gasp, and they both see you.

1. What would you say to Janine?

2. What if the T.A. approaches you and firmly requests that you not tell anyone about what you witnessed, and implies your own grade may be affected if you do?

3. Describe a time where you witnessed or personally faced a conflict of interest.

What type(s) of CASPer scenario is this?

What's the most pressing issue?

What are the missing facts?

Who is directly and indirectly involved?

What are some possible solutions using if/then strategy?

CASPer Scenario 6:

You and your partner are busy lawyers but are taking a much-awaited vacation together. You have outsourced all planning to a travel agent. Upon arrival at your destination, you finally have time to review the itinerary she has put together. To your surprise, the travel agent made reservations in all the wrong restaurants, many of which are out of your budget. She also scheduled tours in places you are not interested in seeing, despite you indicating your preferences to her months before. Her invoice is sitting in your email inbox and you have not yet made any payment to the travel agency.

1. How would you proceed in this situation?

2. What if all the reservations she made, none of which appeal to you, are non-refundable and unchangeable?

3. Describe a time when something for which you had high expectations fell through.

<u>What type(s) of CASPer scenario is this?</u>

<u>What's the most pressing issue?</u>

What are the missing facts?

Who is directly and indirectly involved?

What are some possible solutions using if/then strategy?

CASPer Scenario 7:

While volunteering at a food pantry in your hometown, you meet a refugee from a war-torn country who is your age. Over the months, you spend increasingly more time together, and you learn about the unimaginable difficulties he faced under the country's former repressive regime. You become very close friends. One day, he confides in you that he is in the country illegally, and that he uses a fake document to work and help support his family. The authorities are now investigating him, and he needs you to help vouch for his fake identity.

1. How will you react to your friend's request knowing that if you don't vouch for him, he is likely to get deported and face prosecution in his home country?

2. How should governments create and enforce immigration policies?

3. Describe an ethical dilemma you have faced and how you dealt with it.

What type(s) of CASPer scenario is this?

1. ethical

What's the most pressing issue?

① Legal consequences from the doc

②

What are the missing facts?

What is the document? → maybe it is legal & my friend is unaware cuz diff in his country

How long?

How did he get in knowing strict border agents?

Who is directly and indirectly involved?

D: Myself, my friend's well being

I: My friend's family, society by losing worker. Other ppl that potentially got in w/ same documen

What are some possible solutions using if/then strategy?

If Legal → OK

If not legal → private convo, explain the serious consequences it gets unco-vered. Encourage to turn themselves in would cause the less harm to both of us. If he refuses ⇒ I would have to report him OR speak an authority, although I understand his situation.

We could speak to a lawyer first, knowing my limit-ations.

145

CASPer Scenario 8:

You are visiting your grandfather in the hospital. Your grandfather shares a room with another patient, a man in his 70s. When the nurse comes in to bring this patient food, you see him caressing her, and complimenting her "velvety smooth skin." The nurse is left visibly uncomfortable and leaves the room as soon she can. You witness repeated similar interactions throughout the course of the day every time the nurse comes in to care for the patient.

1. How would you act in this situation?

2. As a witness, is it your responsibility to intervene? Why or why not?

3. Have you ever witnessed or personally experienced a situation where professional boundaries were crossed?

What type(s) of CASPer scenario is this?

What's the most pressing issue?

What are the missing facts?

Who is directly and indirectly involved?

What are some possible solutions using if/then strategy?

CASPer Scenario 9:

You live in a rural community with a high rate of childhood obesity. In most neighboring communities, the youth are avid soda drinkers. One of the soda companies has taken the initiative to sponsor exercise-related events in town. They have organized multiple runs, half-marathons, and even a dance competition. In each event, the company distributes educational pamphlets on the importance of exercise to be fit and healthy.

1. Do you find this company's initiatives problematic? Why or why not?

2. If you were the doctor in town, and were asked to publicly endorse the company's message and the events they sponsored, what would you do?

3. In your opinion, what is the most efficient way to curtail childhood obesity?

What type(s) of CASPer scenario is this?

What's the most pressing issue?

What are the missing facts?

Who is directly and indirectly involved?

What are some possible solutions using if/then strategy?

CASPer Scenario 10:

Many prestigious universities secure part of their spots in each class for legacy admissions. Some argue that these elite colleges exploit admissions as a fundraising tool, as they bring in children of affluent donors who may not have the scores or overall caliber required of other applicants. In fact, many prominent political figures have been accused of "buying their way" into an Ivy League education. You are the Dean of Admissions at your school and you are asked by the school's president to admit two applicants with prominent father figures using the legacy admissions policy.

1. What will you do in this situation?

2. What are the advantages and disadvantages of preferentially admitting legacy students?

3. In your view, what are the most important factors to consider in university admissions?

What type(s) of CASPer scenario is this?

What's the most pressing issue?

What are the missing facts?

Who is directly and indirectly involved?

What are some possible solutions using if/then strategy?

CASPer Scenario 11:

You are a senior doctor at the hospital seeing patients with your resident, who is originally from India. One of your patients has been difficult and occasionally disrespectful to staff throughout his stay. As you go into his room, the resident communicates to the patient he will have to stay in the hospital an extra day due to a delay with his MRI scan. The patient suddenly explodes and yells at the resident: "Your kind is always so incompetent! Go back to your country. We don't want you here. Nurse! Can I please see a real doctor from around here?"

1. As the senior physician, how do you react? What if you were a junior physician?

2. What if you were aware that this patient is very wealthy, and has previously made important donations to the hospital?

3. Have you witnessed acts of discrimination in your life? If so, how have you dealt with them?

What type(s) of CASPer scenario is this?

What's the most pressing issue?

<u>What are the missing facts?</u>

<u>Who is directly and indirectly involved?</u>

<u>What are some possible solutions using if/then strategy?</u>

CASPer Scenario 12:

You are at a lecture by a heart surgeon who has done many international medical missions. In his presentation, he boastfully discusses the wide range of procedures he did while in Africa, including many outside his scope of practice. One student raises her hand and asks if he had received formal training in all the surgeries he performed while abroad. "No, but it was either me or no one else taking out that appendix. At least I knew my way with the scalpel."

1. What are your thoughts on this heart surgeon's actions?

2. If the patients had been made aware of the surgeon's inexperience, would it change your answer?

3. In a world where medicine is increasingly global, what are important things to consider as healthcare professionals?

What type(s) of CASPer scenario is this?

What's the most pressing issue?

What are the missing facts?

Who is directly and indirectly involved?

What are some possible solutions using if/then strategy?

Bonus CASPer scenario:

You are the director of research ethics and you discover that the researchers trusted with creating a new computerized admissions screening tool for prospective professional school candidates, have been falsifying and withholding key findings. There are allegations that the research group is intentionally doing this for economic gains as they seek to commercialize this tool and sell it to other universities.

1. What would you do in this situation and what are the greater implications of such actions, if you kept quiet?

2. You find that the researchers have been lying to both applicants and admissions deans that it is not possible to prepare for their test in hopes of selling their screening tool to more schools who are worried about impact of coaching. What will you do? Do you believe applicants that want to prepare for their tests are better applicants or not?

3. While the school prides itself in being able to select highly ethical and professional candidates, you find out that the school's director of medical education has been writing commentaries for a major national newspaper and the director's comments appear to be one-sided, divisive and discriminatory against a specific group of individuals. What would you do?

What type(s) of CASPer scenario is this?

What's the most pressing issue?

What are the missing facts?

Who is directly and indirectly involved?

What are some possible solutions using if/then strategy?

CASPer Practice Test Two

CASPer Scenario 1:

You are a brain surgeon who recently performed a life-saving operation for a patient. Weeks later, you are flipping through a gossip magazine when you see a picture of your patient walking his daughter down the aisle. You had not realized his daughter was famous. A paragraph in the article is dedicated to your patient's illness, and he is quoted saying: "I am forever grateful to my doctor, who saved my life. Without him, I would not be here today." You are touched and decide to buy the magazine and take it home.

1. Would you show the article to your family and friends?

2. What if a few weeks later, your patient sends you a thank you card in the mail with a copy of the magazine? Would that change your answer to the previous question?

3. Should doctors take additional precautions when their patients are famous? Why or why not?

What type(s) of CASPer scenario is this?

What's the most pressing issue?

What are the missing facts?

Who is directly and indirectly involved?

What are some possible solutions using if/then strategy?

CASPer Scenario 2:

You are on a long flight to Japan. An obese woman weighing about 250 pounds is sitting next to you. Throughout the flight, you are constricted to half your seat, and have no access to the armrest you share with that passenger. You are usually able to sleep during flights, but this trip is very uncomfortable, and you spend all sixteen hours awake. You have an important meeting when you arrive in Japan.

1. Would you say anything to the passenger next to you? Why or why not?

2. If you were a member of the airplane crew, and this was brought to your attention, what would you do?

3. In your view, how should the airline industry respond to an increasingly obese population?

What type(s) of CASPer scenario is this?

What's the most pressing issue?

What are the missing facts?

Who is directly and indirectly involved?

What are some possible solutions using if/then strategy?

CASPer Scenario 3:

You work for a pharmaceutical company, overseeing a clinical study on a new drug for Alopecia Areata. Alopecia Areata is an autoimmune disorder that causes baldness. Patients enrolled in the study receive the drug for free and come in for monthly blood tests. One day, you notice a participant's blood test has a minor abnormality. This patient received tremendous benefit from the drug, and recently left her house without a wig for the first time. Unfortunately, this abnormal blood test makes her ineligible to continue the study. When you inform her of this, she starts crying and begs you not to document this finding. This drug has changed her life dramatically, and she feels she may spiral into a serious depression if it's taken away from her.

1. What would you do in this situation, knowing that this abnormal blood test is likely insignificant?

2. If you were told that the penalty for lying in a clinical trial is incarceration, would that change your actions?

3. Is it better for pharmaceutical companies to be structured as for-profit or non-profit ventures? Please explain your rationale.

What type(s) of CASPer scenario is this?

What's the most pressing issue?

What are the missing facts?

Who is directly and indirectly involved?

What are some possible solutions using if/then strategy?

CASPer Scenario 4:

Many groundbreaking scientific and medical advances were due to animal testing. For example, we owe our understanding of the nervous system to experiments with squids; and treatments for cancer, diabetes, smallpox, and polio were all tested in animals before deemed safe for humans. Generally, our perception of an animal's intelligence decides if they are part of our moral circle, and thus if we can use them in the lab, or even eat them. However, there is a growing body of evidence that suggests animals think, perceive, and feel in ways we did not understand before.

1. What are your views on animal testing?

2. Recently, compelling data came out that shows pigs are as cognitively complex as dogs and chimpanzees —yet society treats them quite differently. If you were a political leader, would you act on this knowledge? If so, how?

3. Throughout history, cultural shifts have drastically affected our perceptions of morality and our behavior as human beings. What is the most significant cultural shift of the last century in your opinion?

<u>What type(s) of CASPer scenario is this?</u>

<u>What's the most pressing issue?</u>

What are the missing facts?

Who is directly and indirectly involved?

What are some possible solutions using if/then strategy?

CASPer Scenario 5:

You are a senior in high school, and you play in the school's volleyball team. The coach's daughter, Marianne, is one of your classmates and also plays on the team. Since you both started high school, she has been the team captain every year. The coach chooses the team captain. Marianne is kind, mature, and an excellent player. You are also a strong player and liked by your peers.

1. Are this coach's actions problematic? If so, how?

2. If you also wanted to be team captain, how would you go about it?

3. Under what circumstances, if any, is it okay for a person in a position of power to appoint family members or friends to other leadership positions?

What type(s) of CASPer scenario is this?

What's the most pressing issue?

What are the missing facts?

Who is directly and indirectly involved?

What are some possible solutions using if/then strategy?

CASPer Scenario 6:

In 1989, a nonprofit organization was created in the United States to address the shortage of teachers and disparity among public schools. This organization recruits thousands of high-performing college graduates to teach in low-resource, often neglected public schools around the country. Graduates serve in the position for two years.

1. What are the benefits and limitations of such a program?

2. If you were given 10 million dollars to address any issue in the public education system in your community, how would you spend this money?

3. How have your own educational opportunities influenced your career decisions?

What type(s) of CASPer scenario is this?

What's the most pressing issue?

What are the missing facts?

Who is directly and indirectly involved?

What are some possible solutions using if/then strategy?

CASPer Scenario 7:

You are a summer volunteer at a clinic in Guatemala. You are supervised by a senior volunteer from your home institution, who traveled with you. This volunteer is an avid blogger and writes daily about his experience at the Guatemalan clinic. When you read his blog, you notice a very paternalistic tone in describing local infectious diseases that have been eradicated in your home country. He does not include any patient identifiers, but you find the text all around disrespectful and condescending.

1. What would you do in this situation?

2. Describe a time when you entered a conflict with someone who was supervising you.

3. What does cultural competency mean to you?

What type(s) of CASPer scenario is this?

What's the most pressing issue?

What are the missing facts?

Who is directly and indirectly involved?

What are some possible solutions using if/then strategy?

CASPer Scenario 8:

You are an undergraduate student working in a research lab. You have been working closely with a senior graduate student as well as your research supervisor. After a year of sleepless nights and many experiments you finally have enough data to start writing a manuscript. You have multiple meetings with your supervisor and the senior graduate student to help guide you with writing your first scientific manuscript. You write your first draft and the manuscript is ready for submission. To your surprise when the final draft is ready for submission you notice that you are second author while the senior graduate student is the first author. Based on conversations with your supervisor you were under the impression that you would be the first author given that you have completed most of the experiments and wrote the manuscript.

1. What is going through your mind?

2. How would you approach this situation?

3. What would you do if you were the principle investigator?

What type(s) of CASPer scenario is this?

What's the most pressing issue?

What are the missing facts?

Who is directly and indirectly involved?

What are some possible solutions using if/then strategy?

CASPer Scenario 9:

You are the supervisor. You work with a married couple. They have been having more heated arguments at the work place over household responsibilities. In particular, the wife notes that she is forced to do all of the housework and feels that the husband is not pulling his weight. The husband says that he has to take care of their son and that takes up the majority of his time. Their arguments are getting to the point that it is now disturbing the work place and impacting their work.

1. You have been tasked to mediate this situation as the supervisor. What would you do?

2. Who do you think is at fault?

3. What suggestions would you have moving forward with workplace arguments that pertain to one's personal life?

What type(s) of CASPer scenario is this?

What's the most pressing issue?

<u>What are the missing facts?</u>

<u>Who is directly and indirectly involved?</u>

<u>What are some possible solutions using if/then strategy?</u>

CASPer Scenario 10:

You visit your favorite restaurant and decide to grab a drink at the bar first before being seated. You notice that the bartender is one of your little sister's friends. Your sister is only 16 and you are concerned that the restaurant is hiring someone under aged.

1. How would you address this situation?

2. What would you do if your sister's friend told you that she needs to make some extra cash to help pay for medical bills for her family member?

3. Under what circumstances should under aged children be allowed to work?

What type(s) of CASPer scenario is this?

What's the most pressing issue?

What are the missing facts?

Who is directly and indirectly involved?

What are some possible solutions using if/then strategy?

CASPer Scenario 11:

Your best friend called you and asked to meet over dinner to discuss something. Turns out he is $25,000 in debt after making some bad investment decisions. He is borrowing money from a "pay-day" loan centre and is paying a very high interest rate. Your friend said he met with the bank and they said they would agree to lend him money at a lower interest rate, but he needs a co-signer. He asks you to co-sign the loan for him and promises to pay everything off now.

1. Would you agree to co-sign for your friend to get the loan? Why or why not?

2. How would you recommend for him to get his finances back in order?

3. Do you think finances and friendship should go together? Why or why not?

<u>What type(s) of CASPer scenario is this?</u>

<u>What's the most pressing issue?</u>

What are the missing facts?

Who is directly and indirectly involved?

What are some possible solutions using if/then strategy?

CASPer Scenario 12:

You are working in a group of five on a collaborative research project. Each member of the group has been assigned a section of the paper to write. The group has been working well together and the paper had seemed to come along great. The group is sending around the paper for a final review the night before it's due to be handed in. When it is your turn to review the paper, you realize that large portions of the paper from other sections which you did not write seem to be plagiarized. It is late at night and you are due to hand in the paper first thing in the morning so there really is no time to rewrite.

1. What do you do in this situation?

2. What if your group members didn't own up to plagiarism?

3. What if your group members insisted on handing the paper in as is?

What type(s) of CASPer scenario is this?

What's the most pressing issue?

What are the missing facts?

Who is directly and indirectly involved?

What are some possible solutions using if/then strategy?

Even more practice: Perfect practice makes perfect!

The best way to truly polish your skills is by doing realistic timed simulations followed by expert feedback. After you have studied this book, go to https://bemoacademicconsulting.com/casperprep to enroll in one of our CASPer prep programs and take advantage of:

1. The only realistic CASPer simulations created by former CASPer raters and scientists proven to increase your practice score by up to 23%.

2. Personalized one-on-one expert feedback to identify your weaknesses and learn how to do better.

3. CASPer prep video course to learn how to ace any type of CASPer question. Note that the contents of the video course are very similar to the content of the book but it may help you if you prefer to watch a video rather than read a book.

4. Access to your typed responses. This will allow you to review your timed responses so you can learn from your mistakes.

5. Numeric scoring of your test just like the real test. Our CASPer experts will score your responses the same way your actual test is scored so you might get an idea of your potential score on the real test.

6. Join the revolution. Your investment supports our development of a brand new, fair and technologically advanced admissions tool.

7. 100% satisfaction guarantee. We offer this for two reasons: a) we want to make sure that we take the risk away from you because we know once you give us a try you are going to love our services and you will choose us as your long term mentors, and b) we wouldn't want to create any program that we wouldn't feel confident offering to our own family and friends at full price.

If you are serious about acing your CASPer test and becoming an excellent future professional, we're serious about helping you. But we have a limited number of spots available because we have a limited number of consultants and we want to maintain the quality of our services. So act now by securing your spots before it's too late by visiting the link below:

https://bemoacademicconsulting.com/casperprep

CHAPTER X

Bonus Resources and Free Sample Test

Here are additional resources to help you prepare for your test:

Free sample practice test:
https://bemoacademicconsulting.com/free-sample-casper-sim-practice-test

BeMo's private CASPer test prep MasterMind Facebook Group:
https://www.facebook.com/groups/BeMo.CASPerTestPrep.MasterMind/

BeMo's Ultimate Guide to CASPer including sample questions, videos, expert analysis, and pro tips: https://caspertestprep.com/

BeMo's Ultimate Pre-Med Resource Center:
https://bemoacademicconsulting.com/premed-resources

BeMo's CASPer prep blog:
https://bemoacademicconsulting.com/blog/category-casper-test.html